T0264324

Palliative Care

Editors

ALAN R. ROTH
SERIFE ETI
PETER A. SELWYN

PRIMARY CARE:
CLINICS IN OFFICE PRACTICE

www.primarycare.theclinics.com

Consulting Editor
JOEL J. HEIDELBAUGH

September 2019 • Volume 46 • Number 3

ELSEVIER

1600 John F. Kennedy Boulevard • Suite 1800 • Philadelphia, Pennsylvania, 19103-2899

http://www.theclinics.com

PRIMARY CARE: CLINICS IN OFFICE PRACTICE Volume 46, Number 3
September 2019 ISSN 0095-4543, ISBN-13: 978-0-323-68241-1

Editor: Jessica McCool
Developmental Editor: Laura Fisher

© **2019 Elsevier Inc. All rights reserved.**

This periodical and the individual contributions contained in it are protected under copyright by Elsevier, and the following terms and conditions apply to their use:

Photocopying
Single photocopies of single articles may be made for personal use as allowed by national copyright laws. Permission of the Publisher and payment of a fee is required for all other photocopying, including multiple or systematic copying, copying for advertising or promotional purposes, resale, and all forms of document delivery. Special rates are available for educational institutions that wish to make photocopies for non-profit educational classroom use. For information on how to seek permission visit www.elsevier.com/permissions or call: (+44) 1865 843830 (UK)/(+1) 215 239 3804 (USA).

Derivative Works
Subscribers may reproduce tables of contents or prepare lists of articles including abstracts for internal circulation within their institutions. Permission of the Publisher is required for resale or distribution outside the institution. Permission of the Publisher is required for all other derivative works, including compilations and translations (please consult www.elsevier.com/permissions).

Electronic Storage or Usage
Permission of the Publisher is required to store or use electronically any material contained in this periodical, including any article or part of an article (please consult www.elsevier.com/permissions). Except as outlined above, no part of this publication may be reproduced, stored in a retrieval system or transmitted in any form or by any means, electronic, mechanical, photocopying, recording or otherwise, without prior written permission of the Publisher.

Notice
No responsibility is assumed by the Publisher for any injury and/or damage to persons or property as a matter of products liability, negligence or otherwise, or from any use or operation of any methods, products, instructions or ideas contained in the material herein. Because of rapid advances in the medical sciences, in particular, independent verification of diagnoses and drug dosages should be made.

Although all advertising material is expected to conform to ethical (medical) standards, inclusion in this publication does not constitute a guarantee or endorsement of the quality or value of such product or of the claims made of it by its manufacturer.

Primary Care: Clinics in Office Practice (ISSN: 0095-4543) is published quarterly by Elsevier Inc., 360 Park Avenue South, New York, NY 10010-1710. Months of issue are March, June, September, and December. Periodicals postage paid at New York, NY and additional mailing offices. Subscription prices are $246.00 per year (US individuals), $505.00 (US institutions), $100.00 (US students), $303.00 (Canadian individuals), $572.00 (Canadian institutions), $175.00 (Canadian students), $357.00 (international individuals), $572.00 (international institutions), and $175.00 (international students). Foreign air speed delivery is included in all *Clinics* subscription prices. All prices are subject to change without notice. POSTMASTER: Send address changes to *Primary Care: Clinics in Office Practice*, Elsevier Periodicals Customer Service, 11830 Westline Industrial Drive, St. Louis, MO 63146. Customer Service Health Sciences Division, Subscription Customer Service, 3251 Riverport Lane, Maryland Heights, MO 63043. **Customer Service: 1-800-654-2452 (U.S. and Canada); 314-447-8871 (outside U.S. and Canada). Fax: 314-447-8029. E-mail: journalscustomerservice-usa@elsevier.com (for print support); journalsonlinesupport-usa@elsevier.com (for online support).**

Reprints. For copies of 100 or more, of articles in this publication, please contact the Commercial Reprints Department, Elsevier Inc., 360 Park Avenue South, New York, NY 10010-1710. Tel. 212-633-3874; Fax: 212-633-3820; E-mail: reprints@elsevier.com.

Primary Care: Clinics in Office Practice is covered in *MEDLINE/PubMed (Index Medicus)* and *EMBASE/ Excerpta Medica, Current Contents/Clinical Medicine,* and *ISI/BIOMED.*

Contributors

CONSULTING EDITOR

JOEL J. HEIDELBAUGH, MD, FAAFP, FACG
Clinical Professor, Departments of Family Medicine and Urology, University of Michigan Medical School, Ann Arbor, Michigan

EDITORS

ALAN R. ROTH, DO, FAAFP, FAAHPM
Chairman, Department of Family Medicine, Ambulatory Care, and Community Medicine, Chief, Palliative Care Medicine, Director, Hospice and Palliative Medicine Fellowship Program, Jamaica Hospital Medical Center, Jamaica, New York

SERIFE ETI, MD
Associate Professor, Department of Family and Social Medicine, Medical Director, Palliative Care Service, Montefiore Medical Center, Albert Einstein College of Medicine, Bronx, New York

PETER A. SELWYN, MD, MPH
Professor, Chair, Departments of Family and Social Medicine, Department of Epidemiology and Population Health, Medicine, Department of Psychiatry and Behavioral Science, Director, Palliative Medicine Program, Montefiore Medical Center, The University Hospital for the Albert Einstein College of Medicine, Bronx, New York

AUTHORS

OLUMUYIWA O. ADEBOYE, MBBS, MBA, FACP, FAAHPM
Medical Director, Palliative Care, Ascension Wisconsin, Ascension St. Elizabeth Hospital Campus, Appleton, Wisconsin

CAITLIN N. BARAN, MD
Attending Physician, Division of Geriatrics and Palliative Care, Massachusetts General Hospital, Harvard Medical School Instructor of Medicine, Boston, Massachusetts

ANGELO R. CANEDO, PhD, MS, LNHA, FACHE
Vice President, MediSys Health Network, Jamaica Hospital Medical Center, Jamaica, New York

FRANK CHESSA, PhD
Director of Clinical Ethics, Maine Medical Center, Assistant Professor of Medicine, Tufts University School of Medicine, Portland, Maine

OSCAR CORZO, MD
Faculty, Palliative Care Department, Jamaica Hospital Medical Center, Jamaica, New York

SERIFE ETI, MD
Associate Professor, Department of Family and Social Medicine, Medical Director, Palliative Care Service, Montefiore Medical Center, Albert Einstein College of Medicine, Bronx, New York

ELIZABETH FIGURACION, DO
Faculty, Palliative Care Department, Jamaica Hospital Medical Center, Jamaica, New York

JOETTE ELISE GREENSTEIN, DO, FAAHPM
Medical Director, Vitas Healthcare, Clinical Associate Professor of Family Medicine, Ohio University Heritage College of Osteopathic Medicine, Dublin, Ohio

ANDY LAZRIS, MD, CMD
Medical Director, Personal Physician Care, Columbia, Maryland

VANESSA LEWIS RAMOS, MD
Assistant Professor, Department of Family and Social Medicine, Palliative Care Service, Montefiore Medical Center, Albert Einstein College of Medicine, Bronx, New York

JOHN LIANTONIO, MD
Assistant Professor, Department of Family and Community Medicine, Division of Geriatric Medicine and Palliative Care, Thomas Jefferson University Hospital, Philadelphia, Pennsylvania

SALLY E. MATHEW-GEEVARUGHESE, DO
Faculty, Palliative Care Department, Jamaica Hospital Medical Center, Jamaica, New York

KATHLEEN MECHLER, MD
Assistant Professor, Department of Family and Community Medicine, Division of Geriatric Medicine and Palliative Care, Thomas Jefferson University Hospital, Philadelphia, Pennsylvania

SHEERA MINKOWITZ, MD, MBA
Fellow, Division of Pediatric Hematology/Oncology, The Children's Hospital at Montefiore, Bronx, New York

LINDA R. MITCHELL, MD
Fellow, Hospice and Palliative Medicine Fellowship, Department of Family and Social Medicine, Montefiore Medical Center, The University Hospital for the Albert Einstein College of Medicine, Bronx, New York

FERNANDO MORENO, MD
Department of Family Medicine and the Division of Palliative Medicine, Maine Medical Center, Medical Director, Hospice of Southern Maine, Clinical Assistant Professor of Family Medicine, Tufts University School of Medicine, Portland, Maine

SARAH NORRIS, MD, MEd
Director of Pediatric Palliative Care and the Quality in Life Team, Children's Hospital at Montefiore, Bronx, New York

JOEL S. POLICZER, MD, FACP, FAAHPM
Senior Vice President of Medical Affairs, Vitas Healthcare, Miramar, Florida; Assistant Adjunct Professor of Medicine, Florida International University Herbert, Wertheim College of Medicine, Miami, Florida

ALAN R. ROTH, DO, FAAFP, FAAHPM
Chairman, Departments of Family Medicine, Ambulatory Care, and Community Medicine, Chief, Palliative Care Medicine, Director, Hospice and Palliative Medicine Fellowship Program, Jamaica Hospital Medical Center, Jamaica, New York

JUSTIN J. SANDERS, MD, MSc
Attending Physician, Department of Psychosocial Oncology and Palliative Care, Dana-Farber Cancer Institute, Harvard Medical School Instructor of Medicine, Boston, Massachusetts

KATHRYN SCHARBACH, MD, MS
Assistant Professor of Pediatrics, Icahn School of Medicine at Mount Sinai, New York, New York

PETER A. SELWYN, MD, MPH
Professor, Chair, Departments of Family and Social Medicine, Department of Epidemiology and Population Health, Medicine, Department of Psychiatry and Behavioral Science, Director, Palliative Medicine Program, Montefiore Medical Center, The University Hospital for the Albert Einstein College of Medicine, Bronx, New York

ERIC S. SHABAN, MD
Regional Medical Director, Vitas Healthcare, Clinical Instructor, Yale Palliative Care Fellowship, Associate Clinical Professor, Quinnipiac University Frank H. Netter MD School of Medicine, Middlebury, Connecticut

NIDHI SHAH, MD
Assistant Professor, Program Director, Hospice and Palliative Medicine Fellowship, Department of Family and Social Medicine, Montefiore Medical Center, The University Hospital for the Albert Einstein College of Medicine, Bronx, New York

E. ALESSANDRA STRADA, PhD, MSCP
Licensed Clinical Psychologist, Palliative Care and Integrative Medicine, Consultant, Faculty, Psychopharmacology Program, Alliant University, San Francisco, California

Contents

Palliative care is a field of medicine that delivers patient-centered care for individuals and their families suffering from serious illness at all stages of the disease trajectory. It addresses the major priorities of relieving suffering, establishing goals of care, and managing physical symptoms while integrating the psychosocial, cultural, spiritual, and existential complexities of coping with chronic illness. This article discusses the role of palliative care in the health care system. It reviews the importance of prognostication, disease trajectory, and communication. The role of the primary care physician as part of a multidisciplinary team member delivering primary palliative care is emphasized.

Hospice is a model of care that offers significant benefits to patients at the end of their lives, their families, and also to the primary care physicians who have diligently cared for their patients. As comprehensive care physicians, primary care physicians can benefit from a strong understanding of hospice and the Medicare Hospice Benefit. This article describes the history of hospice, palliative care versus hospice care, clinical appropriateness of the hospice patient, the regulatory guidelines of the Medicare Hospice Benefit, hospice reimbursement, primary care reimbursement, and employment opportunities in hospice.

The intent of this article is to help clinicians to have practical knowledge and skills related to both assessment and pharmacotherapy of chronic pain in the seriously ill patients. Treating patients with chronic pain and progressive disease should include assessment of "total pain" (physical, psychological, and spiritual suffering) and the care givers as part of treatment team. Effective management of chronic pain starts with thorough assessment and diagnosis of the pain syndrome. A worldwide consensus endorses use of multimodal approach and opioid pharmacotherapy as the mainstay approach to moderate to severe pain in cancer and pain associated with serious illness.

The burden of nonpain symptoms such as anorexia, constipation, nausea, and vomiting contribute to patient suffering throughout the course of advanced illness. It is important to address symptom control throughout the disease trajectory, and especially at the end of life. Primary care clinicians must recognize these symptoms early, provide ongoing assessment, and keep abreast of evidence-based management strategies, including valid clinical protocols.

Primary care clinicians face difficult conversations with patients across the life cycle. As clinicians care for patients in different health states, the focus of these challenging conversations shifts. Even the most skilled clinicians struggle to find the right words at the right time in these scenarios. This article focuses on communication skills to make difficult conversations easier, whether through assigning a health care proxy, breaking bad news, having conversations about serious illness, or leading a family meeting to discuss goals of care.

Patients with serious illness and their family caregivers face numerous ongoing psychological and social concerns and stressors throughout the disease trajectory. Common challenges relate to the need to manage the disease by making complex and often difficult medical decisions. In addition, the presence of psychological and psychiatric distress, including depression and anxiety, may significantly add to the overall symptom burden for the patient and family caregivers. These challenges negatively impact mood, cognitive function, interpersonal relationships, and medical decision making. If not recognized and adequately addressed, they can seriously undermine coping and resilience, eroding psychological well-being and quality of life.

In caring for dying patients, family medicine practitioners intentionally adopt care plans that affect the manner and timing of death. These decisions are morally weighty. This article provides guidance regarding the ethical and legal appropriateness of practitioner decisions near the end of life. Topics include surrogate decision making, advance care planning, medical nutrition and hydration, double effect, futile care, physician-assisted death, voluntarily stopping eating and drinking, palliative sedation to unconsciousness, and cultural humility.

Sarah Norris, Sheera Minkowitz, and Kathryn Scharbach

Pediatric palliative care and hospice medicine is a field in which a multidisciplinary team assists in the management and treatment of infants, children, and young adults with a serious condition. A therapeutic relationship is created among the team, patients, and their caregivers to address total pain. This encompasses exploration of physical pain, social, spiritual, and emotional pain. Patient-centered and family-centered shared decision-making is paramount when setting and revisiting goals of care with patients and their families. Consider a checklist when faced with a dying patient so that the family and team feel supported.

PRIMARY CARE: CLINICS IN OFFICE PRACTICE

SERIES OF RELATED INTEREST

Clinics in Geriatric Medicine (http://www.geriatric.theclinics.com)
Medical Clinics (http://www.medical.theclinics.com)
Physician Assistant Clinics (http://www.physicianassistant.theclinics.com)

THE CLINICS ARE AVAILABLE ONLINE!
Access your subscription at:
www.theclinics.com

Foreword
Goals of Care, Plans for Life

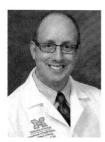

Joel J. Heidelbaugh, MD, FAAFP, FACG
Consulting Editor

In my 20-year career as a family physician, I've been privileged to continue to practice both inpatient and outpatient medicine. I have a loyal panel of patients of all ages, and my practice has been closed to new patients for several years. As many clinicians can attest to, it's tragic when a patient dies, at any age. It is even harder when it is a patient you may have delivered, a coworker, a bandmate, or the most senior member of a multigenerational family. Regardless of the patient, we all hope that we can provide comprehensive and compassionate care for patients and their loved ones at the end of life. What is amazing to realize is that over the last 2 decades, the subspecialty of palliative care has developed and grown into a necessity and fundamental basis of end-of-life care.

This issue of *Primary Care: Clinics in Office Practice* commences with a practical overview of palliative care and hospice principles that can guide primary care clinicians to provide compassionate end-of-life care to patients across the spectrum of age and disease. Articles of management of chronic pain are quite timely, given the national challenges with opiate prescribing juxtaposed with ensuring comfort care. Effective communication with patients and families is paramount, and a skill that takes practice, self-centering, and patience. I found the review of ethical and legal considerations to be very enlightening, and a ready resource for practice. While respect, dignity, and cultural competence remain central to palliative care, religious and spiritual issues should also be respected and valued.

I would like to thank Drs Roth, Eti, and Selwyn as well as the many authors who contributed to this important issue of articles on palliative care. As we strive to provide

Prim Care Clin Office Pract 46 (2019) xiii–xiv
https://doi.org/10.1016/j.pop.2019.06.002
0095-4543/19/© 2019 Published by Elsevier Inc.

compassionate goals of care, perhaps we can also provide biopsychosocial-centered plans for the remainder of life with dignity and grace.

Joel J. Heidelbaugh, MD, FAAFP, FACG
Departments of Family Medicine and Urology
University of Michigan Medical School
Ann Arbor, MI 48103, USA

Ypsilanti Health Center
200 Arnet, Suite 200
Ypsilanti, MI 48198, USA

E-mail address:
jheidel@umich.edu

Preface

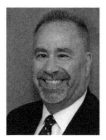
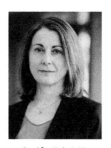
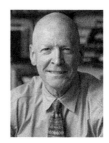

Alan R. Roth, DO, FAAFP, FAAHPM	Serife Eti, MD	Peter A. Selwyn, MD, MPH
	Editors	

Our nation's population is aging, and the cultural and social diversity in our country is steadily increasing. More and more people are suffering with multiple chronic complex illnesses. In addition to this, we have increasing numbers of people who are suffering from functional decline, frailty, debility, and dementia. The complexities of caring for our elderly put an increasing strain on our health care system, and much of this burden is placed on our primary care providers. The need to educate our providers on the care of these individuals is paramount to ensuring the quality of care that our elderly require and deserve for a fulfilling life. It is essential that our primary care providers maintain the continuity of care relationship with the patient and their families. This will ensure that the best possible care is given and that the wishes of our patients are met as they approach the end of life. The scope and practices of the field of Hospice and Palliative Care Medicine are well suited to the work of our primary care providers. Essential skills, such as basic pain and symptom management, communication, prognostication, and advance care planning, are core competencies for all of our primary care clinicians.

The specialty of Hospice and Palliative Care is relatively new and continues to evolve. Emerging evidence is clearly showing that the initiation of palliative care is associated with increased patient and family satisfaction. It helps improve quality of life and assists with difficult decision making. Palliative care helps us improve symptom control and lowers costs.[1,2] The essential goal of palliative care is to help improve and optimize the quality of life for the patient and to support them and their family in navigating the complexities of chronic illness and end-of-life care. Palliative care addresses the major priorities of relieving suffering, establishing goals of care, and managing physical symptoms. It facilitates the integration of the psychosocial, cultural, spiritual, and existential complexities of coping with a chronic complex disease.

The Institute of Medicine[3] 2015 report, "Dying in America: Improving Quality and Honoring Individual Preferences Near the End of Life," clearly documents the need for expanding the utilization and scope of both primary and specialty palliative care. It is essential that the primary care provider maintains an important role in the

Prim Care Clin Office Pract 46 (2019) xv–xvii
https://doi.org/10.1016/j.pop.2019.06.001
0095-4543/19/© 2019 Published by Elsevier Inc.

primarycare.theclinics.com

multidisciplinary approach to care as their patients with chronic complex illness approach the end of life. The role of the specialty palliative care physician should be to augment the care of primary and specialty physicians rather than taking over the care of their patient. Training of primary palliative care skills must become an essential skill taught throughout all phases of medical education. It needs to begin when we are medical students, residents, and fellows and to continue throughout the Attending levels of care.

This issue of *Primary Care: Clinics in Office Practice* is a comprehensive and detailed source of information on palliative care for the student of medicine as well as the practicing clinician. It begins with the introduction of basic palliative care skills, such as pain and nonpain symptom management, and moves forward to highlight the important role of prognostication in formulating goals of care. The issue then addresses more complex domains, such as the psychosocial, ethical issues, and communication skills needed to care for people with serious illness. Additional articles focus on palliative care from the pediatric to the geriatric age group as well as well as a disease-oriented approach to chronic complex illness, such as congestive heart failure, chronic obstruction pulmonary disease, and HIV/AIDS. An article on the role of the primary care provider in hospice care highlights the need for all primary care providers to obtain primary palliative care skills and maintain a continuity of care relationship until the end of life.

Alan R. Roth, DO, FAAFP, FAAHPM
Department of Family Medicine
Ambulatory Care and Community Medicine
Palliative Care Medicine
Hospice and Palliative Medicine
Fellowship Program
Jamaica Hospital Medical Center
8900 Van Wyck Expressway
Jamaica, NY 11418, USA

Serife Eti, MD
Department of Family and Social Medicine
Albert Einstein College of Medicine
Palliative Care Service
Montefiore Medical Center
3347 Steuben Avenue
Bronx, NY 10467, USA

Peter A. Selwyn, MD, MPH
Department of Family and Social Medicine
Palliative Care Program
Montefiore Medical Center
Albert Einstein College of Medicine
3544 Jerome Avenue
Bronx, NY 10467, USA

E-mail addresses:
aroth@jhmc.org (A.R. Roth)
seti@montefiore.org (S. Eti)
selwyn@aecom.yu.edu (P.A. Selwyn)

REFERENCES

1. El-Jawahri A, Greer JA, Temel JS. Does palliative care improve outcomes for patients with incurable illness? A review of the evidence. J Support Oncol 2011; 9(3):87–94.
2. Kavalieratos D, Corbelli J, Zhang D, et al. Association between palliative care and patient and caregiver outcomes: a systematic review and meta-analysis. JAMA 2016;316(20):2104–14.
3. Institute of Medicine. Dying in America: improving quality and honoring individual preferences near the end of life. Washington, DC: The National Academies Press; 2015.

Introduction to Hospice and Palliative Care

Alan R. Roth, DO[a],*, Angelo R. Canedo, PhD, MS, LNHA[b]

KEYWORDS

- Palliative care • Hospice • Multidisciplinary team-based
- Primary versus specialty palliative care • Prognostication • Disease trajectory
- Communication • Advance care planning

KEY POINTS

- Palliative care improves quality of life for patients and their families facing the complexities associated with life-threatening illness through the prevention and relief of suffering.
- Palliative care is most effective early in the course of illness in conjunction with curative care to help manage physical, psychological, and social needs of patients/families.
- The primary care physician who has the trust of the patient/family and an ongoing relationship is well suited to provide primary palliative care.
- Using effective prognostication skills in the care of patients with serious illness fosters the establishment of realistic patient/family focused appropriate goals of care.
- Empathetic communication of prognosis is an essential skill required to care for patients with chronic complex illness, especially as they approach the end of life.

Our nation's population is aging, and people are living with more chronic complex illnesses. These conditions now include augmentative concerns, such as cognitive decline and frailty. The incidence of such concerns is greater than ever before. The number of Americans reaching age 65 and older is projected to more than double from 46 million today to more than 98 million by 2060. These individuals are now approximating 15% of the population, but they will be nearly 24% by the latter part of the century.[1]

Along with the growth of our aging population, the cultural and social diversity of individuals in our country continues to increase. The aforementioned adds a further dimension to the complexity needed for us to deliver patient-centered care, especially

Disclosure Statement: The authors have nothing to disclose.

[a] Department of Family Medicine, Palliative Care Medicine, Hospice and Palliative Medicine Fellowship Program, Jamaica Hospital Medical Center, 8900 Van Wyck Expressway, Jamaica, NY 11418, USA; [b] MediSys Health Network, Jamaica Hospital Medical Center, 8900 Van Wyck Expressway, Jamaica, NY 11418, USA
* Corresponding author. Jamaica Hospital Medical Center, 8900 Van Wyck Expressway, Jamaica, NY 11418.
E-mail address: aroth@jhmc.org

Prim Care Clin Office Pract 46 (2019) 287–302
https://doi.org/10.1016/j.pop.2019.04.001
0095-4543/19/© 2019 Elsevier Inc. All rights reserved.

as these people near the end of life. The demands on our health care system to care for these individuals will put a tremendous burden on providers, and the financial impact will be staggering. Many of these patients with multiple complex illnesses are elderly and account for numerous emergency department and hospital admissions as well as high utilization of intensive care units (ICU). It is estimated that approximately 5% of our patients consume 60% of our health care spending.[2] Much of this is spent on their last year of life and often on their last hospital admission.[3] In addition, the number of individuals living with Alzheimer disease is likely to triple from the current 5 million to nearly 14 million by 2050, adding significantly to costs and caregiver burden.[1]

The Landmark SUPPORT Study that helped define Palliative Care as a specialty was published in 1996. The study highlighted several shortcomings in the delivery of end-of-life care in our country. It noted that only 47% of physicians knew when their patients preferred to avoid cardiopulmonary resuscitation. It found that 46% of do-not-resuscitate orders were written within 2 days of death. Thirty-eight percent of patients who died spent at least 10 days in an ICU. Family members reported moderate to severe pain at least half of the time for 50% of conscious patients who died in the hospital.[4] Unfortunately, in the more than 20 years since the publication of this study, there has not been significant improvement in these statistics. This study emphasizes the need for further enhancements of patient care and medical education in the field of palliative care.

There is some recent evidence that does show positive trends toward more appropriate end-of-life care. The changes especially relate to hospice and ICU utilization. Compared with data from the year 2000, Medicare patients who died in 2015 had a lower likelihood of dying in an acute care hospital. There was also a stabilization of their ICU use during their last month of life. This was accompanied by an increase and then a decline in health care transitions during the last 3 days of life. The decrease in care transitions included a decrease in hospitalizations and transfers from nursing homes.[5]

The utilization of hospice care as well as hospice length of stay has increased as well. This data provides evidence of further improvements in end-of-life care and utilization. Patients who died while receiving hospice care increased from 21.6% in 2000 to 50.4% in 2015. The number who died receiving 3 days or less of hospice care decreased from 9.8% in 2009 to 7.7% in 2015.[5]

The Institute of Medicine 2015 Report, Dying in America: Improving Quality and Honoring Individual Preferences Near the End of Life, clearly documents the state of health care in the United States and the need to increase advance care planning. It also documents the need to expand access to quality palliative care for all. The report highlights the importance of delivering person-centered, family-oriented end-of-life care. It highlights the need for clinician-patient communication, advance care planning, professional education, and development. Consistent with these areas of focus, the report addresses the need for changes in policy and payment systems to support high-quality end-of-life care, public education, and engagement.[6]

There is clear and convincing evidence that palliative care is an effective specialty of medicine. When used early and appropriately, it can assist patients and families with difficult decision making. It also can improve symptom control and lower cost. It can thus effectively improve patient and family satisfaction and possibly even prolong survival.[7,8]

The increased focus on comfort, communication, and the patient-centered team-based approach of palliative care is associated with improved outcomes. This information has been substantiated by data associated with improvements in patient quality of life and family caregiver outcomes. It fosters patient and caregiver satisfaction and improves the quality of care delivered at the end of life.[7,8] A recent meta-analysis published in 2018 reviewed the 6 major studies associated with costs and the utilization of palliative care consultation in hospitalized patients. The study clearly shows significant reductions of cost, which were most notable in patients with cancer, those with significant comorbidities, and when palliative care was initiated within 3 days of the hospital stay.[9] In 2010, studies began to show the benefits of providing palliative care alongside aggressive care. The studies began to look at life expectancy as a result of this intervention. Patients with metastatic non–small cell lung cancer who received palliative interventions along with standard care had significant improvements in both quality of life and mood. The previous individuals also received less aggressive care as they neared the end of life yet also lived longer.[10] Subsequent meta-analysis studies examining survival benefits have failed to substantiate these benefits. However, they do continue to show improved quality of life and lower symptom burden.[8]

The Kaiser Family Foundation published a report in November 2017 titled, "Serious Illness in Late Life: The Public's Views and Experiences." The report reviewed the state of public opinion concerning serious complex illness and end-of-life care. It highlights several facts, including the point that many elderly are aware of the complexities associated with serious illness and are worried about what may happen to them. Only a third of individuals older than the age of 65 have reported talking to their families regarding their concerns and plans about end of life. Only a third have documented their plans in a written document. Of note, very few who have a plan, have shared them with their doctor, thus leading to confusion at end of life.[11] The report once again highlights the need for further education of both the public and the medical profession. Medical professionals need to provide their patients with a better understanding of the complexities associated with chronic illness and the importance of advance care planning and effective communication.

A 2011 public opinion study on palliative care revealed that many patients are worried about their treatment options regarding serious illness. They are concerned about the time and quality of communication with their doctors. Few individuals are aware of the benefits of palliative care, but after being provided with education on the scope of services available, more than 90% of respondents agree that palliative care is important. They state that they would consider it for a loved one, and services should be available for all.[12]

Palliative care is a field of medicine that delivers patient-centered care for individuals and their families. It addresses the suffering for all brought about by serious illness. It can thus be helpful at all stages of the disease trajectory. Palliative care can be helpful at any time after the diagnosis of a life-limiting condition but is often most effective early in the course of the disease in conjunction with curative care, to help manage the physical, psychological, and psychosocial needs of the patients and their families. When cure is no longer possible, relief of suffering becomes predominant and is the foundation of palliative care as both a specialty and a philosophy of care. It is essential that palliative care is differentiated from end-of-life care, which plays a small yet significant role for the palliative care provider (**Fig. 1**).

There are many misconceptions about palliative care, including the belief by many clinicians that palliative care should only be offered when there are no more curative treatments available. In the political arena, palliative care has been associated with death squads and euthanasia. Nothing could be further from the truth. The goal of palliative care is to help improve and optimize the quality of life for the patient. It

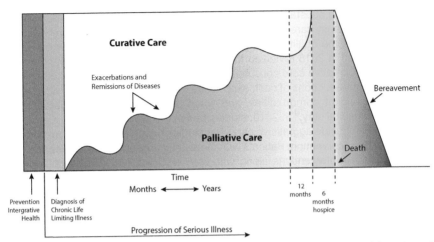

Fig. 1. Continuum of care model for patients with serious illness. (*Adapted from* Lynn J, Adamson DM. Living well at the end of life: adapting health care to serious chronic illness in old age. Santa Monica: RAND; 2003; with permission.)

aims to support patients and their families and to address their complex needs during this difficult time. Effective communication with patients and families helps patients manage the many complex issues they face at this point in life. It helps to restore an appropriate balance between comfort and curative care.

Palliative care uses a multidisciplinary team-based approach to care. It addresses the major priorities of relieving suffering, establishing goals of care, and managing physical symptoms. It also integrates the psychosocial, cultural, spiritual, and existential complexities of coping with a chronic complex disease as one nears the end of life (**Fig. 2**).

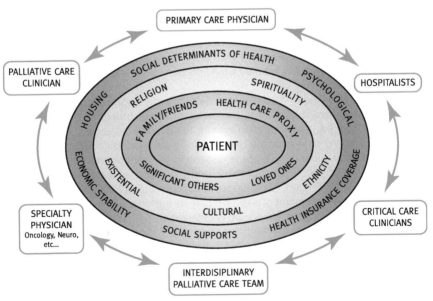

Fig. 2. The complexities of palliative care.

DEFINITIONS

There are many definitions of palliative care, and the World Health Organization definition of palliative care states the following:

Palliative care is an approach that improves the quality of life of patients and their families facing the problem associated with life-threatening illness, through the prevention and relief of suffering by means of early identification and impeccable assessment and treatment of pain and other problems, physical, psychosocial, and spiritual. Palliative care carries out the following:

- Provides relief from pain and other distressing symptoms;
- Affirms life and regards dying as a normal process;
- Intends neither to hasten nor postpone death;
- Integrates the psychological and spiritual aspects of patient care;
- Offers a support system to help patients live as actively as possible until death;
- Offers a support system to help the family cope during the patient's illness and in their own bereavement;
- Uses a team approach to address the needs of patients and their families, including bereavement counseling, if indicated;
- Will enhance quality of life and may also positively influence the course of illness;
- Is applicable early in the course of illness, in conjunction with other therapies that are intended to prolong life, such as chemotherapy or radiation therapy, and includes those investigations needed to better understand and manage distressing clinical complications.[13]

CENTERS FOR MEDICARE AND MEDICAID SERVICES DEFINITION

"Palliative care" means patient- and family-centered care that optimizes quality of life by anticipating, preventing, and treating suffering. Palliative care throughout the continuum of illness involves addressing physical, intellectual, emotional, social, and spiritual needs and to facilitate patient autonomy, access to information, and choice.[14]

Center to Advance Palliative Care Definition

Palliative care is specialized medical care for people with serious illness. This type of care is focused on providing relief from the symptoms and stress of a serious illness. The goal is to improve quality of life for both the patient and the family.

Palliative care is provided by a specially trained team of doctors, nurses, and other specialists who work together with a patient's other doctors to provide an extra layer of support. It is appropriate at any age and at any stage in a serious illness, and it can be provided along with curative treatment.[15]

HOSPICE VERSUS PALLIATIVE CARE

Palliative care is an approach to care for patients and their families that focuses on comfort and quality of life and can be used at any time after the diagnosis of a chronic complex or life-limiting illness. Emphasis is placed on the physical, psychosocial, and spiritual needs of patients. A multidisciplinary team-based approach to care uses primary care and specialty physicians as well as palliative care specialists and a supportive ancillary team. Patients using palliative care do not need to have a terminal diagnosis and may continue to pursue curative therapy, such as chemotherapy and organ transplantation.[16]

Hospice is both a philosophy of care and an insurance benefit that focuses on patients who have a life expectancy of less than 6 months. Patients give up their regular insurance benefit and give up the ability to continue curative therapy and in its place choose aggressive comfort care, which places an emphasis on quality of life rather than quantity and on preparing patients and their families for the end of life. The loss of the ability to continue curative treatments is one of the major barriers to the selection of hospice care.[17] Patients must meet disease-specific criteria and be certified by the primary provider and hospice medical director to have a prognosis of less than 6 months if the disease follows its expected trajectory. The hospice benefit usually includes two 90-day periods followed by an unlimited number of 60-day periods each of which must be certified by the hospice medical director.[18] There are no penalties to patients, families, or providers if the patient outlives the 6-month period. Hospice care is most often given in the home but can also be provided in an inpatient setting, including hospital, nursing home, or stand-alone hospice facilities. Hospice requires a multidisciplinary team-based approach to care and relies on families, friends, and other loved ones as well as volunteers to assist in quality care. Included in the hospice benefit are bereavement services, which assist patient's families for 13 months following the death of the patient.

SCOPE OF SERVICES/DOMAINS OF CARE

Palliative care is rapidly expanding as a specialty in the United States and throughout the world. More than 1700 hospitals currently have palliative care consultation services, and many are now expanding to the ambulatory care setting.[19] Palliative care can be delivered in many settings. In the hospital, there are palliative care consultations services, inpatient units, and ambulatory care programs. Skilled nursing facilities can also offer palliative care consultation services as well as hospice levels of care. Home-based palliative care programs now exist in many communities for patients who continue to pursue aggressive care and are not ready for the transition to hospice (**Box 1**).

Palliative care addresses both pain and nonpain symptom management, but most important, as a field of medicine, requires strong interpersonal and communication skills to address the needs of patients and their families suffering from serious critical illness. Strong prognostication skills are essential to frame difficult discussions related to goals of care, advance care planning, and future treatment plans. Being able to assist in the navigation of the health care system using a team-based approach to care is paramount to successful care and enhanced patient satisfaction.

The identification of which patients are appropriate for palliative care services requires knowledge of the disease trajectory, severity of symptoms and disease burden, and the complex and multifactorial needs of the patient and families. The discussion of when palliative care should be discussed is one of the clinician's most difficult decisions in patient care. An old saying that "it's never too early until it's too late" is most appropriate in the palliative care setting. For this reason, the optimal time for discussion of palliative care services is at the time of diagnosis of chronic complex or serious life-threatening illness (**Box 2**).

TEAM-BASED APPROACH

Palliative care is delivered most optimally and comprehensively when using a team-based approach to care. Because of the complexity of medical, psychosocial, and

Box 1
Domains of palliative care

Assessment and management of pain
  Opioids, nonopioid analgesics, adjunctive pain medications
  Use of cannabinoids
  Rehabilitation, physical therapy, massage
  Interventional pain management
  Psychological approaches (guided imagery, biofeedback)
  Integrative approaches (manual medicine, acupuncture, reiki, meditation)
  Surgery, palliative chemotherapy, and radiation therapy

Nonpain symptom assessment and management
  Dyspnea, nausea, vomiting, diarrhea, constipation, pruritus, hiccups, cough, hemoptysis,
  secretions, mucositis, xerostomia anorexia, cachexia, weight loss, fatigue, fever, lymphedema
  delirium, anxiety, depression, insomnia, anticipatory grief, complicated grief

Prognostication

Assessment of treatment goals of care

Communication skills
  Delivering bad news
  Conducting goals of care family conference

Address spiritual, religious, existential, and cultural aspects of care

Psychosocial issues

Advance care planning discussions
  Health care proxies, surrogate decision maker, durable power of attorney for health care
  Living wills, medical directives, POLST/MOLST forms

Determination of decision-making capacity

Discussions surrounding informed consent/shared decision making

Assessment and treatment of palliative care emergencies
  Impending spinal cord compression, airway obstruction, superior vena cava syndrome,
  intractable pain, cardiac tamponade, massive hemorrhage, hypercalcemia, seizures,
  intestinal obstruction, urinary retention, deep venous thrombosis, and pulmonary embolism

Care of the actively dying patient

Discussing issues related to artificial hydration and nutrition (AHN) including the insertion of
PEG tubes

Palliative procedures
  Paracentesis, thoracentesis, interventional pain management, malignant wound care

Withdrawal and withholding treatments
  Mechanical ventilation, noninvasive positive pressure ventilation
  Dialysis, AHN, automatic implantable cardioverter-defibrillator

The use of palliative sedation

Medical futility or other ethical and legal complexities

Interdisciplinary team assessment and care coordination

Assure continuity of care across settings

Discharge planning and disposition

Bereavement

Box 2
Patients appropriate for palliative care

Anyone with a prognosis of less than 3 years

Advanced chronic complex serious medical illness
    Congestive heart failure, chronic obstructive pulmonary disease, end-stage liver disease
    End-stage renal disease before starting and for those on dialysis
    Advanced, noncurable or metastatic cancer at the time of diagnosis
    Neurodegenerative disorders: dementia, amyotrophic lateral sclerosis, Parkinson disease,
    advanced HIV/AIDS
    Status post cardiac arrest/anoxic brain injuries
    Serious trauma and fractures in advanced age
    Significant head trauma, intracerebral hemorrhage, or strokes

Critically ill patients, those requiring prolonged ICU care, or return to ICU from floor level care

Care of the actively dying patient
    Elderly patients with increased dependence, frailty, debility, failure to thrive, or pressure
    injuries

Patients with multiple comorbidities

Uncontrolled pain or other nonpain symptoms

Patients with frequent emergency department visits and hospitalizations or readmissions

Patients with developmental and intellectual disabilities

Potential organ donor or recipient candidates

Requests for hastened death, euthanasia, or physician-assisted suicide

Homebound, nursing home, or hospice patients

Poor functional or performance status or recent significant decline

Conflicts in medical decision making or patient and family conflict about treatment decisions

Medical futility or other ethical and legal complexities

---

spiritual issues, significant time is needed to appropriately deliver patient care. Additional time needs to be spent with patients as well as their significant others. Family/significant other meetings to address goals of care and advance care planning can often take hours. The previously stated can be difficult under the current hospital and office-based visit time constraints. The interdisciplinary team works collaboratively to coordinate all aspects of care. They deal with the multiple complexities of chronic illness and dying. They need to be especially adept at dealing with patient and family suffering. The team approach helps improve care as well as communication between the patient, family, and caregivers. The team approach also provides a benefit to the caregivers. It affords them a forum for supporting each other. The team members may often be dealing with their own family and self-care issues. Their personal, emotional, and psychosocial care needs coincide with their work in dealing with patients and families who have serious illness and may be facing death (**Box 3**).

PRIMARY VERSUS SPECIALTY PALLIATIVE CARE

With the aging of our population and individuals living longer with chronic complex illness along with a greater acceptance of hospice and palliative care in general, there is a current and projected severe nationwide shortage of palliative care

Box 3		
The interdisciplinary team		
Patient, family, and friends	Social workers	Clinical
Primary care physician	Psychologists	pharmacologists
Specialty physicians	Dietitians	Music/art therapy
Hospitalists	Chaplains	Administrators
Critical care clinicians	Physical therapists	Ethics consultant
Palliative care consultants	Occupational therapy, speech, and	Community health
Physicians assistants and nurse	language pathologists	workers
practitioners	Physical medicine and rehabilitation	Volunteers
Nurses	Wound care specialists	

providers. The current US supply of hospice and palliative medicine (HPM) specialists is inadequate. Given the current training of 325 hospice and palliative fellows each year, it is estimated that there will be a pool of professionals that will range from 8100 to 19,000. Simultaneously, it is estimated that the United States will require up to 24,000 physicians to meet our nation's needs in the future.[20] It is thus clear that to meet the needs of our patients, one must rely on specialty HPM physicians and to meet the needs of the patients one must rely on primary care as well as specialty clinicians to provide primary palliative care services. All clinicians must be trained in basic principles of palliative care. They must be afforded training in essential palliative care clinical skills. The skills should include basic pain and symptom management, psychosocial support, accurate prognostication, and the communications skills needed for advance care planning. Clinicians must be provided with hands-on skills needed to provide patients and their significant others with unwelcomed news and in some cases bad news. They must be trained in how to conduct patient/family meetings wherein they will present and help define the goals of care.

The primary care physician who has the trust of the patient and family as well as a continuing relationship is well suited to provide basic palliative care. The best place to address the complexities brought about by a serious chronic illness is in the setting of the primary care physician's office. A nonemergent setting is optimal for these discussions. Referral for specialty palliative care may be necessary for more complex pain and symptom management. Specialty palliative care can also provide skilled intervention to address severe psychosocial distress, discussions about conflicting goals of care as well as addressing family conflict. Optimal patient outcomes occur when the primary care provider continues as an integral member of the multidisciplinary team even when specialty services are needed.

PROGNOSTICATION

The cornerstone of care in patients with chronic complex illness is the establishment of realistic patient- and family-focused appropriate goals of care. A prognosis is a prediction of possible future outcomes of a treatment or a disease course based on medical knowledge and experience.[21] To establish appropriate goals of care, it is essential to formulate a prognosis that is as accurate as possible. Patients and their families may then be able to set reasonable expectations of care and prioritize what is important to them during the course of their illness. Prognostication helps patients begin to think seriously about end of life and afford themselves insights into their dying. It assists in the patient and significant other decision-making process and facilitates clinicians in their decision making. Patients and families want to know the prognosis because plans will differ greatly if the prognosis is days, weeks, months, or years. Being able to establish a prognosis of less than 6 months is necessary to determine hospice eligibility for most Medicare and Medicaid beneficiaries. A late referral to hospice care is sometimes related to delays in formulating an accurate prognosis. This result may make it more difficult for patients and families to make difficult decisions about their treatment goals until very close to the end of life. Again, an earlier introduction to palliative care allows for time to plan for end of life.

Acquiring appropriate prognostication skills is essential for both the primary care physician and the palliative care specialist. What is formally known as the clinician prediction of survival when used alone has been shown to be inferior to standard prediction models used in palliative care.[22,23] Most studies show that physicians are accurate in survival predictions in only 20% of cases. They will most often overestimate prognosis. This occurs in more than 60% of the cases. This inaccuracy is even greater if the clinician has a closer relationship with the patient. This is often described as primary or general physician bias. It has been demonstrated to overestimate survival by 3- to 5-fold.[24] This inaccuracy has a negative impact on patient and family communication, trust, and the setting of appropriate goals of care.

Accurate prognostication requires a thorough patient evaluation, which includes a complete history and physical examination. The process includes an analysis of prior treatment successes and failures, a review of laboratory and other diagnostic studies as well as discussions with primary care, specialty, and critical care clinicians. Enabling patients and families to establish appropriate and attainable goals is best achieved by integrating several components. These components include a discussion of the natural progression of all diseases as well as specific disease trajectory models. Integrating prior treatments and the utilization of general indicators of health and disease-specific prognostication tools along with sound clinical judgment will help solidify prognostication accuracy.

Subsequently, all medical decision making should be guided by the established care goals and, as the illness progresses, goals will frequently change based on the changing clinical condition and therefore changes in prognosis. The fluctuating course of medical illness, which limits the sensitivity of accurate prognostication, is one of the major challenges associated with selecting patients that are appropriate for palliative care. To be as accurate as possible, the clinician must be educated on the art and science of prognostication. Unfortunately, this important skill has not been emphasized in modern clinical medicine, research, and education.[21] Meticulous clinical judgment using all available information, the clinical picture, and an accurate assessment of the patient's reasonable goals of care is essential for the formulation of an as accurate prognosis as possible.

THE DYING TRAJECTORY

The dying trajectory refers to changes in health status over time as a patient approaches death. The dying trajectory is an important component of prognostication. A century ago, most people died suddenly and often unexpectedly from acute illnesses, such as infections, or from accidents or childbirth. With advances in medical science, individuals are living longer and suffering from multiple complex medical illnesses. Some diseases, such as cancer, take a more predictable course with a steady decline over the last months of life. The chronic organ failure trajectory in progressive conditions, such as congestive heart failure and chronic obstructive pulmonary disease, are more difficult to predict because the disease is associated with repeated exacerbations and remissions.[25] Each decompensating event will often lead to a hospitalization or emergency department visit with the patient not returning to the same functional level as before the illness. The difficulty with these conditions is that it is often never known which episode will lead to a terminal event. Those suffering from dementia or the frail elderly suffer from a slow but steady decline over several years and will sometimes have a sudden demise from cardiac events, infections, or falls. A limitation of the dying trajectory model is that many patients with serious illness often have multiple comorbidities, and many conditions may be associated with sudden death, such as the patient with cancer with a hypercoagulable state suffering a pulmonary embolism (**Fig. 3**).

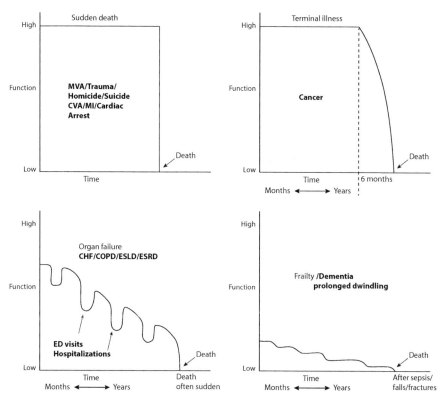

Fig. 3. Proposed trajectories of dying. CHF, congestive heart failure; COPD, chronic obstructive pulmonary disease; CVA, cerebrovascular accident; ESLD, end-stage liver disease; ESRD, end-stage renal disease; MI, myocardial infarction; MVA, motor vehicle accident. (*Adapted from* Lynn J, Adamson DM. Living well at the end of life: adapting health care to serious chronic illness in old age. Santa Monica: RAND; 2003; with permission.)

FUNCTIONAL ASSESSMENT

The assessment of performance status and functional ability has been studied extensively in palliative care and has been shown to be the single most important predictor of survival. There are numerous scales that have been developed, including the Karnofsky performance status (KPS), the palliative performance scale (PPS), and the Eastern Cooperative Oncology Group–Performance Status (ECOG-PS). The PPS is an advancement of the KPS and evaluates ambulation, level of activity, evidence of disease, ability for self-care, oral intake, and level of consciousness. The scale has been shown to have good overall interrater reliability as well as being a useful predictor of mortality.[26,27] The ECOG-PS is an important scale that uses similar parameters and is used extensively by oncologists to determine prognosis, disease progression, and the appropriateness of further cancer treatments, including surgery, chemotherapy, or radiation therapy.[28] Each tool is important for monitoring functional decline as the patient's condition worsens and is a strong prognostic predictor of survival. Decreases in appetite and the ability to eat especially when combined with a weight loss of greater than 10% is a specific and compelling separate indicator of survival. When combined with patient- and disease-specific data, functional assessment is an essential tool in managing all patients as they approach the end of life.

LABORATORY CHANGES

Monitoring of basic laboratory tests as patients chronic conditions worsen may be helpful in conjunction with other clinical data in estimating prognosis. Elevations of calcium, B-type natriuretic peptide, white blood cell counts, as well as inflammatory markers, such as C-reactive protein, are helpful in documenting worsening of disease. Anemia as well as deterioration of liver function and renal function can be helpful as a general indicator of worsening of health.[29] Decreases in cholesterol and albumin are seen commonly as patients deteriorate and are good indicators of declining nutritional status. An albumin of less than 2.5 or rapidly decreasing levels indicate a declining prognosis. A study of frail elderly revealed that a lipid level of less than 160, associated with a decrease in hemoglobin and albumin, was associated with an 84% 1-year mortality versus a 7% mortality in those with normal laboratory findings.[30] Laboratory studies, especially when trended over time, are a helpful resource when used along with functional assessment and disease-specific scales.

COMMUNICATING PROGNOSIS

Patient and family engagement using shared decision making is the cornerstone of effective patient care. The communication skills required to coordinate care for the complex needs of patients with advanced chronic illness is paramount to improved quality of life as well as patient and family satisfaction. Being able to empathetically communicate prognosis is an essential skill needed for all primary and specialty physicians who care for patients with chronic complex illness especially as they approach the end of life. Communicating news related to serious illness as well as death and dying is one of the most difficult tasks for all clinicians. The communication skills needed for delivering bad news and conducting a goals-of-care family meeting is a tool that must be taught at all levels of medical education. There is clearly a need for improved communication between patients, families, and providers. Numerous studies of end-of-life patients and their families show that improved communication is clearly related to enhanced patient and family satisfaction with their care.[7,8] Patients prefer direct and empathetic communication that is neither overly optimistic nor overly pessimistic and includes a practical exchange of information so that the most appropriate decisions can be made. Patient-centered, goal-oriented shared decision making is the cornerstone of effective communication at the time of diagnosis of complex serious medical illness. Numerous benefits of effective communication include encouraging healing relationships, more accurate exchange of information, and better management of uncertainty.[31] There are numerous barriers to effective communication, including culture, religion, spirituality, unrealistic expectations, lack of experience with death and dying, and a lack of trust in the health care system.[32] Personal goals as one approaches end of life often vary greatly and can sometimes be conflicting. It is essential to elicit what is most important to the patient. Is it the longest quantity of life versus the best quality of life, to be pain and symptom free and surrounded by loved ones? Honest, explicit, and open discussions with patients and families concerning their values, hopes, fears, burdens, and treatment preferences will best enable the establishment of realistic and attainable goals of care (**Fig. 4**).

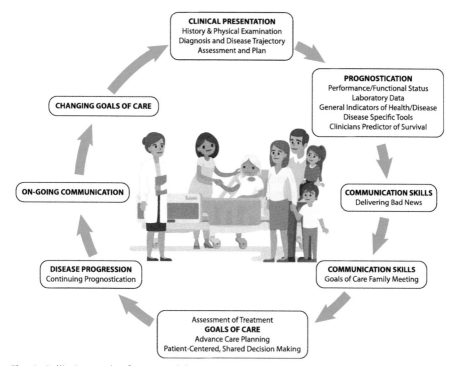

Fig. 4. Palliative goals of care model.

ADVANCE CARE PLANNING

Advance care planning is making decisions about the care you would want to receive if you become unable to speak for yourself. The decisions are yours to make, regardless of what you choose for your care, and the decisions are based on your personal values, preferences, and discussions with your loved ones. Advance care planning involves getting information of what types of life-sustaining treatments are available and deciding what kind of treatments are best for you should you be diagnosed with a life-limiting illness.[33] It is then essential that you share your decisions with your loved ones and ensure that they understand your wishes should you not be able to speak for yourself. It is essential to appoint a health care proxy or surrogate decision maker to make decisions for you if you cannot make them for yourself. The final step is putting this information into a written document that clearly expresses your wishes. Assigning a decision maker by completing a health care proxy or durable power of attorney for health care will ensure the correct person is making decisions for the patient. A written advance directive form, such as a living will or medical directive, should specify what type of treatment a patient does or does not want as they progress through the disease trajectory of chronic serious life-limiting illness. A Physicians Orders for Life Sustaining Treatment (POLST)/ Medical Orders for life Sustaining Treatment (MOLST) form is an actionable medical directive that clarifies what types of life-sustaining treatment are desired at the end of life. This type of document is most appropriate in the last years of life. Medicare and other insurance companies now reimburse physicians for advance care planning in the office and hospital setting. The encounter must be face to face with the patient or their surrogate decision maker. The advance care document does not need to be completed but requires documentation of the discussion regarding the patient's wishes and future treatment desires. There are numerous resources for advance care planning, including "The Conversation Project,"[34] "Respecting Choices,"[35] and the "Serious Illness Conversation Guide"[36] to name a few. Primary care providers who have long-term continuity and trustful relationships with patients and their families are best suited to assist in the advance care planning discussion.

SUMMARY

As noted, listening to a person's thoughts and wishes may lead us to learn that there might be a fate worse than death, such as to live in pain, to suffer alone, to be a burden to others, and especially, to live without dignity. Palliative care is a philosophy of medicine and a medical specialty aimed at meeting the complex needs of patients and families at the most difficult times of their lives. The palliative approach to care addresses the major priorities of relieving suffering, managing physical and emotional symptoms, and establishing realistic goals of care. Palliative care focuses on the psychosocial, cultural, spiritual, and existential complexities of chronic complex serious medical illness as one nears the end of life. Strong prognostication skills need to be accompanied by effective and empathetic communications skills. The physician needs to engage patients and families using patient-centered shared decision making. These components are essential and become the cornerstone of effective patient care. The overall goal of palliative care is to improve the patient's, significant other's, and family's quality of life by using an individualized comprehensive and multidisciplinary approach to care. Primary care physicians play an essential role in the delivery of essential palliative care services. It is crucial that the primary care provider remains an integral part of the team, even when there is a need to augment the service with a specialty level of providers. As a team, they maintain oversight throughout the disease trajectory, including hospice, end-of-life care, and bereavement.

REFERENCES

1. Available at: https://www.prb.org/aging-unitedstates-fact-sheet. Accessed July 15, 2018.
2. Blumenthal D, Abrams MK. Tailoring complex care management for high-need, high-cost patients. JAMA 2016;316(16):1657–8.
3. Aldridge MD, Kelly AS. The myth regarding the high cost of end-of-life care. Am J Public Health 2015;105(12):2411–5.
4. A controlled trial to improve care for seriously ill hospitalized patients. The study to understand prognoses and preferences for outcomes and risks of treatments (SUPPORT). The SUPPORT Principal Investigators. JAMA 1995;274(20):1591–8.
5. Teno JM, Gozolo P, Trivedi AN, et al. Site of death, place of care, and health care transitions among us medicare beneficiaries, 2000-2015. JAMA 2018;320(3): 264–71.

6. IOM (Institute of Medicine). Dying in America: improving quality and honoring individual preferences near the end of life. Washington, DC: The National Academies Press; 2015.

7. El-Jawahri A, Greer JA, Temel JS. Does palliative care improve outcomes for patients with incurable illness? A review of the evidence. J Support Oncol 2011;9(3): 87–94.

8. Kavalieratos D, Corbelli J, Zhang D, et al. Association between palliative care and patient and caregiver outcomes: a systematic review and meta-analysis. JAMA 2016;316(20):2104–14.

9. May P, Normand C, Cassel JB, et al. Economics of palliative care for hospitalized adults with serious illness: a meta-analysis. JAMA Intern Med 2018;178(6):820–9.

10. Temel JS, Greer JA, Muzikansky A, et al. Early palliative care for patients with metastatic non-small-cell lung cancer. N Engl J Med 2010;363:733–42.

11. Available at: https://www.kff.org/report-section/serious-illness-in-late-life-the-publics-views-and-experiences-executive-summary. Acessed August 12, 2014.

12. Available at: https://media.capc.org/filer_public/3c/96/3c96a114-0c15-42da-a07f-11893cca7bf7/2011-public-opinion-research-on-palliative-care_237.pdf. Accessed August 12, 2018.

13. Available at: http://www.who.int/cancer/palliative/definition/en/, Accessed July 15, 2018.

14. Available at: https://www.cms.gov/Medicare/Provider%85and%85/Survey-and-Cert-Letter-12-48. Accessed July 28, 2018.

15. Available at: https://www.capc.org/payers-policymakers/what-is-palliative-care. Accessed August 12, 2018.

16. Available at: https://www.nia.nih.gov/health/what-are-palliative-care-and-hospice-care. Accessed October 8, 2018.

17. Finestone AJ. Inderwies G Death and dying in the US: the barriers to the benefits of palliative and hospice care. Clin Interv Aging 2008;3(3):595–9.

18. Available at: https://www.medicare.gov/Pubs/pdf/02154-Medicare-Hospice-Benefits.PDF. Accessed October 8, 2018.

19. Available at: https://www.capc.org/topics/hospital/. Accessed October 8, 2018.

20. Lupu D, Quigley L, Mehfoud N, et al. The growing demand for hospice and palliative medicine physicians: will the supply keep up? J Pain Symptom Manage 2018;55(4):1216–23.

21. Christakis N. Death foretold: prophecy and prognosis in medical care. Chicago: University of Chicago Press; 1990.

22. Hui D, Park M, Liu D, et al. Clinician prediction of survival versus the palliative prognostic score: which approach is more accurate? Eur J Cancer 2016;64: 89–95.

23. Farinholt P, Park M, Guo Y, et al. A comparison of the accuracy of clinician prediction of survival versus the palliative prognostic index. J Pain Symptom Manage 2018;55(3):792–7.

24. Christakis NA, Lamont EB. Extent and determinants of error in doctors' prognoses in terminally ill patients: prospective cohort study. Br Med J 2000;320:469–73.

25. Murray SA, Kendall M, Boyd K, et al. Illness trajectories and palliative care. BMJ 2005;330(7498):1007–11.

26. Campos S, Zhang L, Sinclair E, et al. The palliative performance scale: examining its inter-rater reliability in an outpatient palliative radiation oncology clinic. Support Care Cancer 2009;17:685.

27. Harold J, Rickerson JT, McGrath J, et al. Is the palliative performance scale a useful predictor of mortality in a heterogeneous hospice population? J Palliat Med 2005;8(3):503–9.

28. Oken MM, Creech RH, Tormey DC, et al. Toxicity and response criteria of the Eastern Cooperative Oncology Group. Am J Clin Oncol 1982;5:649–55.

29. Reid VL, McDonald R, Nwosu AC, et al. A systematically structured review of bio-markers of dying in cancer patients in the last months of life; an exploration of the biology of dying. PLoS One 2017;12(4):e0175123.

30. Vedery RB, Goldberg AP. Hypocholesterolemia as a predictor of death: a pro-spective study of 224 nursing home residents. J Gerontol 1991;46(3):M84–90.

31. Wright AA, Zhang B, Ray A, et al. Associations between end-of-life discussions, patient mental health, medical care near death, and caregiver bereavement adjustment. JAMA 2008;300(14):1665–73.

32. Kagawa-Singer M1, Blackhall LJ. Negotiating cross-cultural issues at the end of life: "you got to go where he lives". JAMA 2001;286(23):2993–3001.

33. Available at: https://www.nhpco.org/advance-care-planning-. Accessed October 8, 2018.

34. Available at: http://theconversationproject.org/. Accessed October 8, 2018.

35. Available at: https://respectingchoices.org/. Accessed October 8, 2018.

36. Available at: https://www.ariadnelabs.org/areas-of-work/serious-illness-care/. Ac-cessed October 8, 2018.

Hospice for the Primary Care Physician

Joette Elise Greenstein, DO[a,b,*], Joel S. Policzer, MD[c,d], Eric S. Shaban, MD[e]

KEYWORDS

- Hospice • Primary care physician • Hospice admission criteria
- Medicare hospice benefit

KEY POINTS

- Primary Care physicians can benefit from a strong understanding of hospice and the Medicare Hospice Benefit by learning the regulations of the benefit and how hospice providers are reimbursed.
- As a comprehensive caregivers, primary care physicians should understand the clinical appropriateness of a hospice patient to ensure a timely referral to hospice.
- Collaborative care is a major importance in the care of hospice patients, and primary care physicians will benefit from understanding their relationship with hospice providers.
- Primary care physicians can be reimbursed for the care they provide to their hospice patients and should understand how to correctly bill for their services.

Hospice is a model of care that offers significant benefits to patients at the end of their lives, their families, and also to the primary care physicians (PCPs) who have diligently cared for their patients. As comprehensive care physicians, PCPs can benefit from a strong understanding of hospice and the Medicare Hospice Benefit (MHB). This article describes the history of hospice, palliative care versus hospice care, clinical appropriateness of the hospice patient, the regulatory guidelines of the MHB, hospice reimbursement, primary care reimbursement, and employment opportunities in hospice.

HISTORY OF HOSPICE

Hospices and the hospice movement have a long history and tradition that go back to the eleventh century. At that time, Crusaders opened refuges for travelers. The name "hospice," deriving from the Latin *hospes*, connotes the host and the guest. These

Disclosure: The authors have nothing to disclose.
[a] Vitas Healthcare, 655 Metro Place South, Suite 770, Dublin, OH 43017, USA; [b] Ohio University Heritage College of Osteopathic Medicine, 6775 Bobcat Way, Suite 230, Dublin, OH 43016, USA; [c] Vitas Healthcare, 3046 Corporate Way, Miramar, FL 33025, USA; [d] Florida International University, Herbert Wertheim College of Medicine, Miami, FL, USA; [e] Vitas Healthcare, 199 Park Road Extension, Suite 102, Middlebury, CT 06762, USA
* Corresponding author. Vitas Healthcare, 655 Metro Place South, Suite 770, Dublin, OH 43017.
E-mail address: Joette.greenstein@vitas.com

Prim Care Clin Office Pract 46 (2019) 303–317
https://doi.org/10.1016/j.pop.2019.04.002
0095-4543/19/© 2019 Elsevier Inc. All rights reserved.
primarycare.theclinics.com

refuges evolved into places where not only travelers, but the ill and dying, a different form of traveler, could find respite. This type of hospice seemed to languish after The Middle Ages until it was revived in Europe by religious orders specifically created to care for the sick.[1] They were scattered across the continent, run by various orders of nursing sisters, and were in existence until before World War I. The Religious Sisters of Charity opened Our Lady's Hospice in Dublin, Ireland, in 1879, followed by hospices in Australia, and then St Joseph's Hospice in London in 1905, which still exists today.[2]

The modern hospice movement began after World War II and is attributed to Dame Cicely Saunders. Dame Cicely began her career as a registered nurse and medical social worker in Oxford in the 1940s. After caring for a terminally ill man in a long-term setting, she was encouraged to go to medical school. Once she earned her degree in 1957, she began to develop the basic structures of current hospice care based on her experiences at St. Joseph's Hospice: focus on the patient and family, not just the disease.[3] She introduced the concept of "total pain" or "total suffering," where attention was given to the interrelationships of the psychosocial and spiritual needs of the person and the physical symptoms; and the utility of the interdisciplinary team (IDT) in patient care.[4] It has been said that Dame Cicely was a one-person IDT: she was nurse, social worker, and physician. She would not hesitate to clean, bathe, or feed a patient if an aide was not available, and she was able to lead worship on Sunday, if needed (Palliative Care team, St. Christopher's Hospice, personal communication, July, 2003).

Dr Saunders opened St Christopher's Hospice in 1967. A few years later in the early 1970s, Florence Wald, the Dean of the nursing school at Yale, and Edward Dobihal, the Director of Religious Ministries at Yale, began investigating ways to bring Dr Saunders' hospice version to the states. The first American hospice was opened in New Haven, Connecticut in 1974.[5,6]

The MHB was established in 1983. According to the most recent statistics available at the time of this publication, there were just over 4000 hospices in the United States in 2014, and these hospices served 1.43 million patients and families in 2016. In 2016, 48% of Medicare decedents accessed hospice services before their deaths.[5]

PALLIATIVE CARE VERSUS HOSPICE CARE

There is a continuum of palliative care as a patient approaches the end of their disease process. Because Medicare does not have a specific palliative care benefit, PCPs are providing this care. These visits are billed under Medicare Part A or B depending on the location of the visit. If a patient is referred to hospice at the appropriate time (less than 6-month prognosis) then the hospice provides the palliative care under the MHB. Most of hospice care is palliative care until the last days of life when the patient is transitioning to death. Understanding that palliative care is part of the end-of-life continuum helps PCPs refer to hospice sooner.

CLINICAL APPROPRIATENESS

PCPs are at the forefront of identifying patients who are appropriate for hospice care. They remain the primary gateway into the health care system for patients. PCPs manage and co-manage neurologic disease, cardiopulmonary disease, liver disease, renal disease, cancer, and protein-calorie malnutrition into their advanced stages. They are collaborating with oncologists, pulmonologists, nephrologists, and other consultants in their patient's care. As a result, they are an integral part in identifying when their patient is at the end of their disease process. In 2017, the percentage of patients under hospice care by principle diagnosis were as follows:

Cancer	27.2%
Cardiac and circulatory	18.7%
Dementia	18%
Respiratory	11%
Stroke	9.5%
Other	15.6%[7]

Cancer remains the most prevalent diagnosis for hospice patients, representing 27.2% of patients, followed by cardiac disease and dementia. However, noncancer diagnoses comprise most hospice admissions at 72.9%. The principal hospice diagnosis is defined as the diagnosis that has been determined to be the most contributory to the patient's terminal prognosis.

The foremost challenge for PCPs pertains to the timing of the referral to hospice. Most physicians wait too long. In 2017, the average length of service for Medicare patients enrolled in hospice in 2016 was 71 days. The median length of service was 24 days.[7] The causes of late referral are many. As a whole, we live in a society that is "death-denying" and dying is a topic that is simply deflected for as long as possible. There is conventional wisdom that if we talk about dying and eventual death, then we lose focus on current treatments and may actually receive less than optimal treatment. At times, this becomes a self-fulfilling prophecy. So as a result, we defer the conversation for as long as possible because "hospice is where you go to die," even as patients may be actively declining in function. However, eventually the hospice referral becomes inevitable. Patients then progress to advanced debilitation and die quickly once under care, "proving" that hospice is where patients go to die.

Physicians also delay because of the perceived difficulty in determining a patient's limited prognosis. Although tools exist to aid in prognosis, these tools were developed on populations and they are difficult to apply to an individual. Also, physicians tend to overestimate the prognosis of patients with whom they have had a long, therapeutic relationship.[8] One validated tool that is helpful is, "The Surprise Question," which is as follows: would you be surprised to see this patient in your office or clinic 1 year from now? If the answer is "yes," then the patient should be approached about developing an advanced directive that details their long-term goals of care.

Most patients who are entering the advanced stages of their disease process have particular signs and symptoms of decline. They become increasingly dependent on others or require equipment to complete their activities of daily living. Bathing, dressing, ambulation, and transferring are the most common activities of daily living that become affected. For example, in patients with noncancer diagnoses, dependence in three or more of the six activities of daily living meets a criterion for hospice appropriateness.

This decline is specifically detailed in a tool called the Palliative Performance Scale (PPS). The PPS is an 11-point scale designed to measure patients' performance status in 10% decrements from 100% (healthy) to 0% (death) based on five observable parameters: (1) ambulation, (2) ability to do activities, (3) self-care, (4) food/fluid intake, and (5) consciousness level.[9] It is a modified version of the Karnofsky Performance Scale developed to assess patients with cancer, and is typically used by hospice and palliative professionals to describe functional status of a patient. A PPS score of 50 indicates significant disease and functional decline, and a PPS less than or equal to 40 indicates extensive disease and functional decline (**Fig. 1**).

VICTORIA HOSPICE

Palliative Performance Scale (PPSv2)
version 2

PPS Level	Ambulation	Activity & Evidence of Disease	Self-Care	Intake	Conscious Level
100%	Full	Normal activity & work No evidence of disease	Full	Normal	Full
90%	Full	Normal activity & work Some evidence of disease	Full	Normal	Full
80%	Full	Normal activity with Effort Some evidence of disease	Full	Normal or reduced	Full
70%	Reduced	Unable Normal Job/Work Significant disease	Full	Normal or reduced	Full
60%	Reduced	Unable hobby/house work Significant disease	Occasional assistance necessary	Normal or reduced	Full or Confusion
50%	Mainly Sit/Lie	Unable to do any work Extensive disease	Considerable assistance required	Normal or reduced	Full or Confusion
40%	Mainly in Bed	Unable to do most activity Extensive disease	Mainly assistance	Normal or reduced	Full or Drowsy +/- Confusion
30%	Totally Bed Bound	Unable to do any activity Extensive disease	Total Care	Normal or reduced	Full or Drowsy +/- Confusion
20%	Totally Bed Bound	Unable to do any activity Extensive disease	Total Care	Minimal to sips	Full or Drowsy +/- Confusion
10%	Totally Bed Bound	Unable to do any activity Extensive disease	Total Care	Mouth care only	Drowsy or Coma +/- Confusion
0%	Death	-	-	-	-

Instructions for Use of PPS (see also definition of terms)

1. PPS scores are determined by reading horizontally at each level to find a 'best fit' for the patient which is then assigned as the PPS% score.

2. Begin at the left column and read downwards until the appropriate ambulation level is reached, then read across to the next column and downwards again until the activity/evidence of disease is located. These steps are repeated until all five columns are covered before assigning the actual PPS for that patient. In this way, 'leftward' columns (columns to the left of any specific column) are 'stronger' determinants and generally take precedence over others.

   Example 1: A patient who spends the majority of the day sitting or lying down due to fatigue from advanced disease and requires considerable assistance to walk even for short distances but who is otherwise fully conscious level with good intake would be scored at PPS 50%.

   Example 2: A patient who has become paralyzed and quadriplegic requiring total care would be PPS 30%. Although this patient may be placed in a wheelchair (and perhaps seem initially to be at 50%), the score is 30% because he or she would be otherwise totally bed bound due to the disease or complication if it were not for caregivers providing total care including lift/transfer. The patient may have normal intake and full conscious level.

   Example 3: However, if the patient in example 2 was paraplegic and bed bound but still able to do some self-care such as feed themselves, then the PPS would be higher at 40 or 50% since he or she is not 'total care.'

3. PPS scores are in 10% increments only. Sometimes, there are several columns easily placed at one level but one or two which seem better at a higher or lower level. One then needs to make a 'best fit' decision. Choosing a 'half-fit' value of PPS 45%, for example, is not correct. The combination of clinical judgment and 'leftward precedence' is used to determine whether 40% or 50% is the more accurate score for that patient.

4. PPS may be used for several purposes. First, it is an excellent communication tool for quickly describing a patient's current functional level. Second, it may have value in criteria for workload assessment or other measurements and comparisons. Finally, it appears to have prognostic value.

Fig. 1. Palliative Performance Scale (PPSv2). (© Victoria Hospice Society, BC, Canada (2001) www.victoriahospice.org).

In addition to decline in functional status, patients may have unintentional weight loss of more than 10% of normal body weight or a body mass index less than 22.[10] Their disease progression may also result in increased health care use including multiple hospitalizations; emergency room visits; and consultations for physical, occupational, speech therapy, and home health. During these recurrent hospitalizations they show disease progression through laboratory and diagnostic studies and serial physician assessments.[10]

Prognosis can also be determined by the decline within a specific disease process. The following is an overview of determining prognosis in the following disease categories: cardiopulmonary disease, neurologic conditions, end-stage renal disease, end-stage liver disease, end-stage AIDS, cancer, and other common hospice diagnoses. Please note that these are guidelines to be used in evaluating patients. Patients do not need to exhibit all signs and symptoms listed, and the total of their symptom burden from all diagnoses and comorbidities prevails in determining a terminal prognosis.

Cardiopulmonary Disease

Clinical conditions that meet the requirements include but are not limited to congestive heart failure, coronary artery disease, and chronic obstructive pulmonary disease.

Congestive heart failure

This covers patients with New York Heart Association functional class IV (dyspnea at rest despite optimal medical therapy) or New York Heart Association functional class III (dyspnea on minimal exertion despite optimal medical therapy), and the presence of significant comorbidities or secondary conditions. These patients may have preserved

Definition of Terms for PPS

As noted below, some of the terms have similar meanings with the differences being more readily apparent as one reads horizontally across each row to find an overall 'best fit' using all five columns.

1. Ambulation

The items '**mainly sit/lie**,' '**mainly in bed**,' and '**totally bed bound**' are clearly similar. The subtle differences are related to items in the self-care column. For example, 'totally bed bound' at PPS 30% is due to either profound weakness or paralysis such that the patient not only can't get out of bed but is also unable to do any self-care. The difference between 'sit/lie' and 'bed' is proportionate to the amount of time the patient is able to sit up vs need to lie down.

'**Reduced ambulation**' is located at the PPS 70% and PPS 60% level. By using the adjacent column, the reduction of ambulation is tied to inability to carry out their normal job, work occupation or some hobbies or housework activities. The person is still able to walk and transfer on their own but at PPS 60% needs occasional assistance.

2. Activity & Extent of disease

'**Some**,' '**significant**,' and '**extensive**' disease refer to physical and investigative evidence which shows degrees of progression. For example in breast cancer, a local recurrence would imply 'some' disease, one or two metastases in the lung or bone would imply 'significant' disease, whereas multiple metastases in lung, bone, liver, brain, hypercalcemia or other major complications would be 'extensive' disease. The extent may also refer to progression of disease despite active treatments. Using PPS in AIDS, 'some' may mean the shift from HIV to AIDS, 'significant' implies progression in physical decline, new or difficult symptoms and laboratory findings with low counts. 'Extensive' refers to one or more serious complications with or without continuation of active antiretrovirals, antibiotics, etc.

The above extent of disease is also judged in context with the ability to maintain one's work and hobbies or activities. Decline in activity may mean the person still plays golf but reduces from playing 18 holes to 9 holes, or just a par 3, or to backyard putting. People who enjoy walking will gradually reduce the distance covered, although they may continue trying, sometimes even close to death (eg. trying to walk the halls).

3. Self-Care

'**Occasional assistance**' means that most of the time patients are able to transfer out of bed, walk, wash, toilet and eat by their own means, but that on occasion (perhaps once daily or a few times weekly) they require minor assistance.

'**Considerable assistance**' means that regularly every day the patient needs help, usually by one person, to do some of the activities noted above. For example, the person needs help to get to the bathroom but is then able to brush his or her teeth or wash at least hands and face. Food will often need to be cut into edible sizes but the patient is then able to eat of his or her own accord.

'**Mainly assistance**' is a further extension of 'considerable.' Using the above example, the patient now needs help getting up but also needs assistance washing his face and shaving, but can usually eat with minimal or no help. This may fluctuate according to fatigue during the day.

'**Total care**' means that the patient is completely unable to eat without help, toilet or do any self-care. Depending on the clinical situation, the patient may or may not be able to chew and swallow food once prepared and fed to him or her.

4. Intake

Changes in intake are quite obvious with '**normal intake**' referring to the person's usual eating habits while healthy. '**Reduced**' means any reduction from that and is highly variable according to the unique individual circumstances. '**Minimal**' refers to very small amounts, usually pureed or liquid, which are well below nutritional sustenance.

5. Conscious Level

'**Full consciousness**' implies full alertness and orientation with good cognitive abilities in various domains of thinking, memory, etc. '**Confusion**' is used to denote presence of either delirium or dementia and is a reduced level of consciousness. It may be mild, moderate or severe with multiple possible etiologies. '**Drowsiness**' implies either fatigue, drug side effects, delirium or closeness to death and is sometimes included in the term stupor. '**Coma**' in this context is the absence of response to verbal or physical stimuli; some reflexes may or may not remain. The depth of coma may fluctuate throughout a 24 h period.

© Copyright Notice.

The Palliative Performance Scale version 2 (PPSv2) tool is copyright to Victoria Hospice Society and replaces the first PPS published in 1996 [J Pall Care 9(4): 26-32]. It cannot be altered or used in any way other than as intended and described here. Programs may use PPSv2 with appropriate recognition. Available in electronic PDF format by email request to edu.hospice@viha.ca Correspondence should be sent to the Director of Education & Research, Victoria Hospice Society, 1952 Bay Street, Victoria, BC, V8R 1J8, Canada

Fig. 1. (*continued*).

left ventricular function caused by diastolic failure or an ejection fraction less than or equal to 20% caused by systolic failure.[10]

Coronary artery disease

There are patients with structural disease that leads to significant functional impairment with no further medical or surgical interventions either possible or desired. These patients have significant secondary or comorbid conditions, such as symptomatic arrhythmias, history of myocardial infarction, cardiac arrest, and/or syncope.[10]

Chronic obstructive pulmonary disease

This refers to patients with significant impairment in forced expiratory volume in 1 second resulting in dyspnea at rest or with minimal exertion despite optimal medical therapy. These patients are frequently house-confined because of their decline. Requirement of continuous oxygen therapy, frequent episodes of acute shortness of breath, poor response to bronchodilators, either via metered-dose inhalers or nebulization, and presence of cor pulmonale are markers for advanced lung disease.[10]

Neurologic Diseases

Dementia

Patients with such diagnoses as Alzheimer disease, vascular dementia, frontotemporal dementia, and Lewy body dementia may advance to end-stage dementia. The main symptoms of advanced dementia, regardless of cause, present in the following ways: inability to ambulate without assistance, inability to speak or communicate clearly, incontinence of bowel and bladder function, and inability to dress or bathe without assistance. Patients frequently have difficulty swallowing or refuse to eat, requiring diet modifications. Patients may also have related illnesses caused by the dementia including aspiration pneumonia, recurrent fevers, decubitus ulcers, and bacteremia.[10]

Amyotrophic lateral sclerosis

Patients with end-stage amyotrophic lateral sclerosis have rapid progression of the disease and at least one of the following: critically impaired ventilatory capacity that is not responding to ventilator support or refusal of ventilator; life-threatening complications, such as deep decubitus ulcers or significant infections; and critical nutritional impairment with decision not to pursue artificial feeding or poor response/complications with artificial feedings.[10]

End-Stage Renal Disease

This refers to patients with chronic kidney disease Stage V (glomerular filtration rate <15%) who meet the criteria for dialysis and/or renal transplant who refuse the treatment or patients on dialysis who no longer want to continue dialysis.[10] Also included are patients with chronic kidney disease stage 4 (glomerular filtration rate <20%) who have significant symptom burden, such as altered mental status, intractable nausea, intractable hyperkalemia, hepatorenal syndrome, or other significant comorbid diseases.[10]

End-Stage Liver Disease

Patients are considered to be in the terminal stage of liver disease if they meet the following criteria: prothrombin time greater than 5 seconds or international normalized ratio greater than 1.5 and serum albumin less than 2.5 gm/dL, plus one of the following:

  Ascites, refractory to treatment or patient noncompliant
  Spontaneous bacterial peritonitis
  Hepatorenal syndrome
  Hepatic encephalopathy
  Or recurrent variceal bleeding despite treatment

Documentation of progressive malnutrition, muscle wasting with reduced strength and endurance, continued active alcoholism, hepatocellular carcinoma, and hepatitis B or C are also conditions that also meet the criteria.[10]

Human Immunodeficiency Virus Disease

Patients with end-stage AIDS have a CD4 count of less than 25 cells/mm^3 in periods free of acute illness, human immunodeficiency virus RNA (viral load) greater than 100,000 copies on a persistent basis, or less than 100,000 copies in the presence of refusal to take antiretroviral medications, and declining functional status. Other factors associated with poor prognosis include chronic diarrhea for 1 year; persistent serum albumin less than 2.5 g/dL; age greater than 50; congestive heart failure; or the decision to forgo antiretroviral therapy, chemotherapy, and prophylactic medications.[10]

Cancer

Most patients are appropriate for hospice if they have stage IV cancer with presence of metastases that are not responding to treatment or patient elects no further treatment. Stage III cancer may be appropriate if the tumor is causing other comorbid conditions, such as bronchial obstruction, hemorrhage, or if Eastern Cooperative Oncology Group score is greater than 2 because of functional decline (**Table 1**).

Protein Calorie Malnutrition

Malnutrition is used as a terminal diagnosis when weight loss is the major manifestation and it results in a declining PPS score, typically 40% or lower. Studies have shown

Table 1	
Eastern Cooperative Oncology Group performance status	
Grade	**Eastern Cooperative Oncology Group**
0	Fully active, able to carry on all predisease performance without restriction.
1	Restricted physically strenuous activity but ambulatory and able to carry out work of a light or sedentary nature, for example, light house work, office work.
2	Ambulatory and capable of all self-care but unable to carry out any work activities. Up and about more than 50% of waking hours.
3	Capable of only limited self-care, confined to bed or chair more than 50% of waking hours.
4	Completely disabled. Cannot carry on any self-care. Totally confined to bed or chair.
5	Dead

(*From* Oken MM, Creech RH, Tormey DC, et al. Toxicity and response criteria of the Eastern Cooperative Oncology Group. AMJ Clin Oncol 1982;5:649–55; with permission.)

that unintentional weight loss and underweight body mass index (<19) are associated with higher mortality rates among older adults.[10]

Adult Failure to Thrive/Debility

Although adult failure to thrive and debility can no longer be used as a primary terminal diagnosis, they are still valid for determining the patient's overall terminal prognosis and are used as secondary or comorbid conditions. Adult failure to thrive and debility are diagnoses that describe patients with advanced functional decline caused by multiple illnesses present, but none is determined to be the prime reason for the poor prognosis.

Acute Causes of Death

Acute causes of death are diseases that are as advanced or severe as to lead to the patient's imminent demise. Examples of these disease are severe sepsis, aspiration syndrome, heart failure, acute respiratory failure, renal failure, anoxic brain injury, and metabolic encephalopathy.

REGULATIONS FOR HOSPICE ELIGIBILITY

All hospice care is guided by federal regulations published in the Federal Register, updated periodically, and known as the Conditions of Participation. The Conditions of Participation describe how hospices are structured, how care is given and by whom, the responsibilities of the various professionals involved, and how reimbursement is determined.[11]

The Interdisciplinary Team

The IDT is the basic core of how hospice care is given. It derives from the original work of Dame Cicely Saunders and has been written in the federal regulations. Because hospice care focuses on all the domains that affect the patient and family, professionals with expertise in these domains work together to give the care. Physical symptoms and needs are in the domain of the physician and nurse, emotional and social issues are the domain of the social worker, and the chaplain is tasked with addressing spiritual needs.[12,13] Nursing aides are not mandated in the regulations, but many hospices add their expertise to see to the personal hygiene and care of the patients.[14] In the field, it is expected that all the professionals, regardless of discipline, be aware of the patient's total symptoms so that the appropriate care is given. For example, the psychosocial staff is trained to recognize and report any increase in physical symptoms, such as pain or dyspnea, and physicians and nurses should be able to respond to emotional stresses and spiritual issues and bring in additional help as needed.

The team meets at a minimum once every 15 days to review the patients entrusted to them, and to plan the care for the patients for the coming time period. It is expected that all members of the team participate in the care planning, adding in what they know and what they have observed, so that the visits to the patient are appropriate in number and by the needed discipline. At the least, there must be one encounter every 14 days.[13] Usually the nursing aides visit multiple times per week, as does the primary nurse, with physician, social worker, and chaplain visiting as needed.

Prognostication

The prime regulatory role of the hospice centers on prognostication and the certification and recertification of patients as being terminally ill and appropriate for hospice care. The regulations give no guidance as to prognostic criteria, and, in essence, the regulation is that a patient is terminally ill with a prognosis of 6 months or less if the disease follows its expected course and is therefore hospice appropriate as determined by the medical judgment of a Doctor of Medicine or Doctor of Osteopathy.[15]

Over the years, intermediary supervisory organizations, Medicare Administrative Contractors, set up by Centers for Medicare and Medicaid Services have developed Local Care Determinations to assist in prognostication. The latest update has emphasized that patient appropriateness is based on their prognosis not simply their terminal diagnosis. What this means practically is that the sum total of physical changes that the patient has undergone, which will predict, more likely than not, a life-limiting course of 6 months or less. One takes into consideration nutritional status, overall function and the rate at which that function has declined, level of cognition and the rate at which that has declined, the total symptom burden the patient carries from all his or her medical problems and how the total burden adds and accelerates decline, the quantity of health care use, plus specific disease-related criteria.[16] These are used to produce narratives that satisfy the three regulatory tasks a physician must do: (1) certification, (2) recertification, and (3) face-to-face encounter.

Certification

A patient starts their hospice encounter by being referred by a physician who knows the patient, their clinical situation, and goals of care well. Even as the health care system continues to fragment and fewer people have long-term relationships with their physicians, it is usually the PCP that knows the patient best. This is the physician who knows what the patient would want in the face of a severe illness, and can assist in decisions regarding goals of care, such as artificial nutrition, mechanical ventilation, or renal-replacement therapy. This referring physician must sign a certifying document that the patient has a life-limiting illness. It is then the responsibility of the hospice physician, after review of medical records and hospice evaluation, to develop a narrative that explains the patient's decline and why the prognosis is terminal.

A picture needs to be painted to answer the question: "why hospice now?" It is useful to describe function in terms of "the patient could do .... 6 months ago, but now can't, and won't be able to again." A complete narrative includes documentation of nutritional status, cognitive status, functional status, and use of health care.[17]

Recertification

Just as a patient must be certified to access hospice services, the patient must be reevaluated on an ongoing basis to determine that the terminal illness is still present and that the patient remains appropriate for care. Regulations stipulate that there are "benefit periods" for patients' care; the first two are 90 days each, followed by an unlimited number of 60-day periods. At the beginning of each benefit period, recertification must be done that consists of discussion by the IDT of the patient's status, decline in functional status, nutrition, and so forth.

Decline in function, decline in cognition, loss of weight, and worsening of the underlying illness are all factors that are taken into account for recertification. Often subtle factors can support the decision, especially in patients that manifest advanced debilitation. The need for more caregivers to assist in basic tasks is a measure of decline (eg, the patient used to be able to move to a bedside commode, but now it takes two people to assist in repositioning). Additionally, time to task completion is a measure of decline (eg, the patient was able to finish his meal by himself in 15 minutes, but now he must be fed and it takes 40 minutes).

Although laboratory data or imaging do not play a routine role in hospice care, it should be offered if it provides beneficial information that helps the IDT team decide on continued care. For example, a patient was taken under care of hospice with the typical symptoms of cancer of the pancreas, and a scan showed a large mass in the body of the gland but biopsy was refused by the patient. Eight months later the patient continues to do well, with no further weight loss and a reduction in pain. A repeat scan is necessary to document decline. If the mass is present and larger, then this is evidence for the patient to be recertified. If, however, the mass is no longer present, then it may well have been inflammatory, not malignant, and the patient is no longer eligible for hospice care.

All this information is then documented in a recertification narrative by the hospice physician. A hospice patient may be recertified for an unlimited number of benefit periods as long as they continue to have documentation of decline. It should be noted that the referring physician is not required to sign any further prognostic documents after initial certification; the onus is completely on the hospice to develop documentation to support the need for their continued recertification.[17]

Face-To-Face Evaluation

The face-to-face evaluation is a regulatory assessment that was instituted to provide an additional level of certainty that patients who remain under care beyond 6 months meet the criteria of terminal illness. It requires that a physician or advanced practice nurse visit and examine the patient and document their findings that the patient remains terminally ill. This must be done before any recertification starting with the third benefit period. This evaluation does not have to be done by the physician belonging to the team that cares for the patient. Many hospices are able to hire physicians and advanced practice nurses to do this evaluation, and it gives a larger number of clinicians an insight into what hospice care is about; many of them then decide to pursue positions on an IDT.[18]

Hospice Discharge

A patient may be discharged from a hospice for several reasons. The patient may decide to revoke the hospice benefit to seek aggressive treatment. The patient may die, move out of the hospice's service area, or transfer to another hospice. The hospice may determine the patient is no longer terminally ill and discharge the patient for extended prognosis. Additionally, a patient may be discharged for cause if the patient or home environment is such that the delivery of care to the patient or the ability of the hospice to operate effectively is seriously impaired.

If a patient is discharged for extended prognosis or revocation for treatment they can be readmitted at any time if their condition declines and they meet criteria again for certification. However, they do not restart their benefit process from the beginning but instead are admitted in the benefit period following their discharge. For example, if they were discharged in their third benefit period they would be readmitted onto their fourth benefit period. Any patient being admitted after their second benefit period needs a face-to-face evaluation as part of their certification.[19]

HOSPICE REIMBURSEMENT

The MHB was established in 1982 as a comprehensive benefit under Medicare Part A to manage the care of terminally ill patients whose prognosis was 6 months or less through an IDT-oriented approach to care. A key part of the development of the MHB was to establish a hospice payment structure. Under the MHB payment structure, all care required to manage the patient's terminal illness is provided by the hospice. The terminal illness is defined as all conditions that are contributing to the patient's terminal decline including the primary hospice diagnosis plus secondary conditions and any related comorbid conditions.

All unrelated diagnoses are determined by the IDT and care for them is provided to the patient through other parts of Medicare. The Social Security Act, federal regulations, and Hospice Conditions of Participation require hospices to provide medications, biologics, medical equipment, supplies, nursing and nursing aide, social work, spiritual, bereavement, dietary, and therapy services that are related to the hospice plan of care and the palliation and management of the patient's terminal prognosis.

The hospice payment structure consists of four levels of hospice care and professional services that are designed to provide virtually all the patient's care and to support the patient and family through their hospice journey. The four levels of care include (1) routine home care (RHC), (2) continuous home care (CHC), (3) general inpatient care, and (4) intermittent respite care. All four levels of care must be offered by Medicare-certified hospices, and each level of care is based on the clinical needs of the patient. Reimbursement for each level is different and represents the intensity of services that the patient requires to manage their symptom burden.

Routine Home Care

RHC is the most commonly provided level of care for patients receiving hospice services. It represented 98% of the care provided by hospices in 2017, with 56.5% of this being provided in private residences, 42.5% in nursing facilities, and 1% being provided in hospice inpatient facilities and contracted hospitals. This level delivers a comprehensive, interdisciplinary approach to the patient where they reside, including private homes, nursing homes, assisted living facilities, group homes, and retirement communities. Patients receive nursing, nursing aide, chaplain, social work, and physician services in their home in addition to medical equipment and medications related to their terminal illness. This level of care is reimbursed by Medicare through a per diem structure.

The reimbursement of RHC was recently updated in 2016. Hospices are now reimbursed two separate per diem rates for RHC. For Days 1 to 60 there is a higher rate paid because typically patients require more intensive services during the initiation of care. The rate for 2017 set by Medicare was $191 per patient per day. This is the same rate that is paid to all Medicare-certified hospices and is updated annually through the annual hospice wage index from Centers for Medicare and Medicaid Services. Medicare identified that intensity of services declined for patients living beyond 60 days under the care of hospice. Therefore, the RHC rate for days 61+ in 2017 was $150 to provide all of the same services to the patient in their homes. Medicare also recognized that there is an increased clinical and psychosocial need for patients in the last 7 days of life.[20] To account for this Medicare provides a Service Intensity Add-on for registered nurse and social worker visits that occur in the last 7 days of life. This add-on payment is the hourly continuous care rate (described later) multiplied by the number of visits from those disciplines in the last days of life.[21] This payment demonstrates an understanding of the complexities of the dying process and allows hospices to ensure that the needs of the patient and family are met.

Continuous Home Care

CHC is a higher level of hospice care that is available to patients who have increased or increasing symptom burden that requires continuous assessment by a skilled nurse to guide and administer interventions needed to manage the patient. Commonly patients at the end of life experience symptoms of pain, dyspnea, and delirium that are severe and rapidly progressing. These difficult to manage symptoms often require a coordinated interdisciplinary approach to modify the hospice plan of care on an ongoing basis. CHC is provided to patients meeting criteria for a minimum of 8 hours a day up to 24 hours. The care provided should be skilled and provided by a nurse for 51% of the time. The other 49% are provided by a nurse's aide and primary caregiver support. These interventions are initiated from the time that the unmanaged symptoms are identified until they resolve and require a physician's order to start and stop this level of care. CHC is billed by the hospice in 8-hour increments and is reimbursed at an hourly rate of $40.19 to a daily maximum of $965.[22] CHC is intended to be used on a short-term basis to meet the increased care needs of the patient's symptom burden and to rapidly manage the patient's symptoms. Once the symptoms are adequately managed the higher level of care is discontinued and the patient is returned to RHC. Despite this level of care being provided by the MHB, CHC is a level of care that is not commonly used by hospice patients representing only 0.2% of the days of hospice care in 2016.

General Inpatient Care

General inpatient care, like CHC, is another higher level of hospice care that is available to meet the needs of the patient who has increased or increasing symptom burden that cannot be managed in the home setting. This level of care is provided in hospice inpatient facilities. It can also be provided in hospitals or skilled nursing facilities where the hospice contracts with the facility to pay for the bed, staff, and ancillary care to provide and coordinate the patient's plan of care. The goal of this higher level, like CHC, is to rapidly manage the symptoms, stabilize the patient, and transition the patient back home to RHC. This level of care is used the way an acute emergency department visit or hospitalization is used in the nonhospice setting. General Inpatient Care, like CHC, also requires orders to initiate and discontinue care and requires ongoing input from the physician to effectively modify the patient's plan of care. In 2016 the use of this level of care was higher than CHC but still far less than RHC at 1.5% of total days of care provided to beneficiaries.[23] This level of care is reimbursed by Medicare at a daily rate of $724. This higher rate reflects the increased skilled care needs and medical management that the patient would require during these periods of increased symptom burden.[22]

Intermittent Respite Care

The last of the four levels of care to be discussed is intermittent respite care. This level of care is provided for up to 5 consecutive days and is intended to be used to provide respite for the primary caregivers of the patient. Intermittent respite care is provided for the patient in a hospice facility, contracted nursing facility, or contracted hospital. This level of care is reimbursed by Medicare at a $171 per day in 2017.[24] This represents the increased cost of providing care in these inpatients settings because of room and board. This level of care is one of the most infrequently used level of care, only representing 0.3% of all Medicare days for all beneficiaries.[22] This may be related to a median length of service of only 24 days in 2016.

PRIMARY CARE REIMBURSEMENT

There are many questions that arise as patients reach the end of their lives. For example, what is the relationship between the PCP and the hospice? Can the PCP remain involved in the patient's care or does the PCP have to cede control and decision-making over to the hospice? How does the PCP get reimbursed?

The federal regulations of the MHB clearly state that the physician who knows the patient best, the PCP, should continue to be involved in the care of the hospice patient. A hospice offering quality care should encourage the PCP to be involved in their patient's care and make this involvement as easy as possible. This allows a patient to have a smooth transition to hospice with their PCP involved in their end-of-life decisions.

The MHB recognized the importance of professional services at the end of life to ensure high-quality hospice care and effective symptom management. For this reason, the MHB includes a fee-for-service method of billing for employed hospice physicians and nurse practitioners, and for the PCPs who remain the attending physician for the patient.

For physicians and nurse practitioners that are employed with a hospice, the hospice submits a bill to Medicare part A on their behalf. The bills are determined by the practitioner who conducts the visit and are based on location of services and level of complexity of the visit. The Medicare Administrative Contractors reimburse the hospice 100% of the fee schedule for physician visits and 85% for nurse practitioner services. For professional services performed by a provider who performs other functions as a volunteer employee, the hospice must demonstrate that the provider was reimbursed for the professional services that were rendered.[22]

The attending physician is defined as the physician or nurse practitioner most involved in the care of the patient and who was chosen by the patient at the time of hospice election. Attending providers, not associated with the hospice in any way, can also provide professional services for conditions related to the terminal illness; however, the practitioner must submit the bill directly to Medicare part B with the appropriate G modifier to identify how these services relate to the Hospice Benefit. The GV modifier is used for services that are related to the terminal illness. For hospice patients receiving professional services from their Attending provider unrelated to the terminal illness, the GW modifier must be used when submitting the bill. If these modifiers are not used with billing submission, Medicare denies reimbursement. These services are also reimbursed based on location of services and service intensity from the Medicare fee schedule.

If the hospice patient has professional services related to the terminal illness provided by a consulting physician, these services are billed to the hospice directly and reimbursed to the physician. These consultant services by nonhospice or nonattending professionals need to be approved by the Hospice before being rendered in most cases.[22,25]

PRIMARY CARE PHYSICIAN–HOSPICE RELATIONSHIPS

The relationship between the patient's PCP and the hospice staff should be a close and collaborative one. The PCP knows the patient and family best and can advise the hospice on aspects unique to this situation that improve and optimize the care given. For any medical issues that do not relate to the patient's terminal prognosis, the PCP retains the ability to manage, and be reimbursed, for any and all care.

Because it is not expected that the PCP will be able to attend IDT meetings on a regular basis, reports are sent to the physician detailing what discussion was held regarding the PCP's patient and what care plans were instituted or modified. The PCP should review these reports and has the right to contact the IDT manager and hospice physician with any changes or feedback. These reports form an ongoing narrative of hospice care so that the PCP can answer questions and counsel the family if needed.

It should not be the policy or practice of any quality hospice to "take over" the care of patients referred. The attitude should always be one of collaboration, which offers benefits to the PCP, and in turn, to the patients.

The PCP should be able to be involved as much as he or she chooses. If this means that the PCP wants to be called for any and all decisions, then that is what should be done. If the PCP wants to be called during business hours only, with the hospice physicians covering after hours, then that can be put in place, and the PCP should expect updates to the plans of care as they may be changed. If the PCP chooses to obtain reports only, not be involved in day-to-day care, and be informed when the patient dies, that is also a possibility. Although a not infrequent request because of time constraints, it may be perceived by patients and families as a type of abandonment that may adversely affect the patient. It is optimal if PCPs determine some way to let their patients and families know that they remain involved in the care being given and are aware of their patients' status.

In addition, there is always the possibility that the PCP will advance to working with the hospice on a part-time basis, or even transition to a full-time position. Physicians can be on an IDT, managing that census of patients; they can also only come to home visits, work in an inpatient unit, and do face-to-face evaluations and so on.

HOSPICE EMPLOYMENT

Joining a hospice organization is a way of caring for even more patients at the end of life. Physician employment opportunities with hospice organizations vary from per diem to part-time or full-time arrangements with varying levels of clinical and administrative responsibilities. Many hospices employ physicians on a part-time basis to do the Medicare regulatory face-to-face visits that are required for patient's entering their third or higher benefit period.

Clinical visits to home settings to manage symptoms for patients on higher levels of care are another key opportunity in hospice organizations. Additionally, many hospices have hospice inpatient units where they provide the general inpatient level of care for patients with increased symptom burden. Care provided to these patients is often done on a rotation basis by a physician team similar to the way inpatient rounding is provided. Depending on the size of the unit and occupancy, the time commitment varies.

A more involved role that is available to physicians is the role of a hospice team physician. In this role, the physician works as a key part of the interdisciplinary process and development of the hospice plan of care and certification and recertification of the patients. The physician works with the IDT to provide care to a panel of patients in an ongoing basis.

Additionally, the role of hospice medical director is often a mix of clinical, educational, and administrative responsibilities. The hospice medical director is a key leader of the hospice organization whose responsibility is driving and ensuring that high quality of care is being provided to eligible hospice patients, educating the staff and community on the hospice benefit, and working with the hospice program leadership for further development and growth. Depending on the size of the hospice, the hospice medical director position is a part-time or full-time position. A hospice medical director is typically encouraged to pursue their Hospice Medical Director Certification, but this is not required by any federal regulations.

Finally, all hospices must provide twenty-four-hour coverage for their patients and many hospices have the opportunity for physicians to participate in the on-call schedule for their programs. This is often layered into the other positions described, but can also be a stand-alone option with some hospices.

SUMMARY

Many PCPs, both family medicine and internal medicine specialists, find the practice of hospice medicine not depressing, nor hopeless, but the extension of their expertise to give excellent care at the end of life. The care for these patients is meaningful and impactful for the primary care provider and patient. There is a unique sense of satisfaction that is gained by following a patient through the entirety of their illness. It offers the PCP the opportunity for closure, can strengthen physician patient relationships, and helps to promote continuity of care during this important part of a patient's life.

When a physician is present for their hospice patients they can make certain their patients are receiving the care they need, while avoiding care and interventions that are no longer appropriate. By seeing how this improves the time that people have left, it often validates why medicine was the physician's chosen profession in the first place.

REFERENCES

1. Robbins J. Caring for the dying patient and the family. Hagerstown (MD), London: Taylor & Francis; 1983. p. 138.
2. Lewis MJ. Medicine and care of the dying: a modern history. Oxford, England: Oxford University Press US; 2007. p. 20.
3. Poor B, Poirrier GP. End of life nursing care. Hagerstown (MD), London; Boston: Jones and Bartlett; 2001. p. 121.
4. Clark D. Total pain: the work of Cicely Saunders and the hospice movement. APS Bulletin 2000;10(4).
5. Connor SR. Hospice: practice, pitfalls, and promise. Taylor & Francis; 1998. p. 5.
6. NHPCO facts and figures: hospice care in America. Alexandria (VA): National Hospice and Palliative Care Organization; 2018. Rev. ed.
7. The National Hospice and Palliative Care Organization (NHPCO) facts and figures. Alexandria (VA): National Hospice and Palliative Care Organization; 2017 edition.

8. Christakis NA, Lamont EB. Extent and determinants of error in physicians' prognoses in terminally ill patients. West J Med 2000;172(5):310–3.

9. Victoria Hospice Society. Palliative performance scale (PPSv2) version 2. Medical care of the dying. 4th edition. Victoria, (BC): Victoria Hospice Society; 2006. p. 120.

10. Wright JB, Kinzbrunner BM. Predicting prognosis: how to decide when end-of-life care is needed. In: End of life care. New York, NY: McGraw Hill; 2011. p. 5–29. Chapter 1.

11. Available at: https://www.hospiceofthevalley.net/med-pros/eligibility-guidelines.

12. Stajkovic S, Aitken EM, Holroyd-Leduc J. Unintentional weight loss in older adults. CMAJ 2011;183(4):443–9.

13. Conditions of participation for hospice programs; Title 42, Vol 2, Pt 418. 48 Fed.Reg. 56026 (December 16, 1983).

14. Condition of participation: Interdisciplinary group, care planning, and coordination of services. 42 C.F.R. § 418.56. 1983.

15. Condition of participation: core services. 42 C.F.R. § 418.64. 1983.

16. Condition of participation: hospice aide and homemaker services. 42 C.F.R. § 418.76 2009.

17. Condition of Participation: eligibility requirements 42 C.F.R. § 418.20 2005.

18. Medicare Program; FY 2014 hospice wage index and payment rate update; hospice quality reporting requirements; and updates on payment reform," 78 Fed. Reg. 48234-48281 (7 August 2013).

19. Certification of terminal illness. 76 Fed. Reg. 47331 (August 4, 2011).

20. Face to face encounter. 75 Fed. Reg. 70372 (Jan 1, 2011).

21. § 418.26 Discharge from hospice care. 79 Fed. Reg. 50509 (August 22, 2014).

22. Available at: http://www.medpac.gov/docs/default-source/payment-basics/medpac_payment_basics_16_hospice_final.pdf

23. Available at: https://www.gpo.gov/fdsys/pkg/FR-2017-05-03/pdf/2017-08563.pdf

24. Available at: https://www.nhpco.org/sites/default/files/public/Statistics_Research/2017_Facts_Figures.pdf

25. Available at: https://www.cms.gov/Regulations-and-Guidance/Guidance/Manuals/Downloads/clm104c11.pdf. P52

Assessment and Management of Chronic Pain in the Seriously Ill

Vanessa Lewis Ramos, MD, Serife Eti, MD*

KEYWORDS

- Chronic pain • Seriously ill • Opioids • Adjuvant analgesics

KEY POINTS

- Chronic pain requires multidimensional assessment and management.
- Most of the seriously ill patients with chronic pain can be managed adequately by tailoring the regimen to the type of pain syndrome and comorbidities.
- Prescribers should be aware of risk stratification and management to reduce likelihood of problems when prescribing opioids.

INTRODUCTION

Patients with cancer and other life-limiting illnesses may experience chronic pain. About 90% of patients with cancer report pain during their illness trajectory.[1] Dame Cicely Saunders described the concept of total pain, which integrates physical, psychosocial, and spiritual pain.[2] When pain is unrelieved, it can be a source of great distress. It can abate quality of life and decline in physical function and social interaction.[3] Chronic pain also can be psychologically devastating because it can be a constant reminder of the incurable and progressive nature of the disease.[4]

Effective pain management during serious illness is the right of the patient and the obligation of the clinician, as basic analgesic interventions are within the purview of primary care providers. In order to enhance the quality of life of seriously ill patients, clinicians should have primary palliative care skills, which are essential to control pain and nonpain symptoms.[5]

Although education and training have increased for physicians in the management of pain, many patients do not receive adequate analgesia.[6] More than 70% of patients with cancer report pain,[7] and more than 36% of patients with metastatic disease have

Disclosure Statement: The authors have nothing to disclose.
Department of Family and Social Medicine, Palliative Care Service, Montefiore Medical Center, Albert Einstein College of Medicine, 3347 Steuben Avenue, Bronx, NY 10467, USA
* Corresponding author.
E-mail address: Seti@montefiore.org

Prim Care Clin Office Pract 46 (2019) 319–333
https://doi.org/10.1016/j.pop.2019.05.001
0095-4543/19/© 2019 Elsevier Inc. All rights reserved.

primarycare.theclinics.com

pain severe enough to impair function.[8] Pain not only adversely affects the quality of life of patients but also may force otherwise independent individuals to become prematurely institutionalized when they can no longer be managed at home.

The Agency for Health Care Policy and Research (AHCPR), American Pain Society, and the National Comprehensive Cancer Control Program have published comprehensive review of assessment and management of pain guidelines. The prescribers need to be aware of the public health crisis of opioid misuse and consider harm reduction strategies in how they prescribe opioid analgesics, and balance harm prevention with the imperative for relieving suffering.

This article reviews assessment and treatment of chronic pain in the seriously ill and required core competencies for the primary care providers.

ASSESSMENT OF PAIN
Types of Pain and Characteristics

Pain is classified as acute and chronic. Acute pain serves as a protective function but becomes pathologic when no longer serves that function. Chronic pain is defined by the International Association for the Study of Pain as "pain that persists beyond normal tissue healing time, which is assumed to be 3 months."[9] It may be more related to changes in nervous system than to initial tissue injury.[10,11]

There are 3 types of pain: visceral, somatic, and neuropathic. The cornerstone of adequate pain management is a thorough patient assessment including frequent reassessments. A complete history and a physical examination, with emphasis on the patient's symptoms, are obtained, including information regarding the location, intensity, quality, timing, duration, radiation, and aggravating factors.[12]

1. Visceral pain arises from direct stimulation of afferent nerves in the viscera by compression, obstruction, infiltration, ischemia, stretching, or inflammation. This pain tends to be poorly localized, often described as vague. Visceral pain can be deep, aching, squeezing, cramping, or colicky. In patients with cancer, visceral pain may be caused not only by direct tumor infiltration but also by other conditions such as constipation or ileus.[13]
2. Somatic pain is caused by injury to the skin, other soft tissues, bones, or joints. In patients with cancer, it is generally due to soft tissue inflammation or metastatic disease to the bone. Bone pain is thought to be due to either direct stimulation of nociceptors in the periosteum, a release in inflammatory mediators, or an increase in interosseous pressure.[14] It is usually localized, constant, and exacerbated with movement.
3. Neuropathic pain is caused by an injury, lesion, or disease to the peripheral nervous system and central nervous system and is disproportionate to the stimulation of the nociceptor. Clinically, neuropathic pain occurs in an area of sensory deficit.[15] Neuropathic pain can be described as burning, shooting, or electrical, and it is often described as a "pins and needles." Positive symptoms of neuropathic pain include paresthesia and/or dysesthesia, allodynia, hyperalgesia.[16]

The assessment of pain should be multidimensional and specifically targeted to patient population. There are many tools available for pain assessment; however, their use is not well adopted because they are generally perceived as cumbersome.[17] Pain intensity, as reported by the patient, remains the gold standard for pain assessment. The most commonly used pain scales are the numerical rating scale, visual analog scale, and the categorical scale (mild, moderate, severe). In general, numeric scores correspond as 1 to 3: mild, 4 to 6: moderate, and 7 to 10: severe. Pain intensity should be assessed during initial examination and follow-up visits (**Table 1**).

In patients with severe cognitive impairment, observing behavioral cues such as crying, moaning, grimacing, closing eyes tightly, combativeness, and asking family and caregivers will be helpful to determine the extent of pain. When there is doubt, a trial of analgesics is appropriate.[18] Caregivers should be educated to report pain-related behaviors.

Multidimensional Pain Assessment

Effective pain management involves understanding the complex interactions between physiologic, psychological, sociocultural, and cognitive dimensions of pain expression. It is important to properly evaluate the impact of pain on every aspect of the individual's functioning.[19] Pain, and especially cancer pain, is not a pure nociceptive, physical experience but involves different dimensions of the human being, such as personality, affect, cognition, behavior, and social relations. The term "total pain" has been used to characterize multidimensional nature of pain in patients with serious illness.[20] A patient's experience of advanced illness is complex: from suffering physical symptoms to coping, financial concerns, caregiver burden, social and family changes, and spiritual concerns.

A multidimensional pain assessment should include physical, psychological, social, and spiritual domains and involves the following[21]:

1. History and physical examination: cancer history, including recent chemotherapy and/or radiation. Medication reconciliation. Pain characteristics and impact on functional status.

Table 1
Basic pain assessment

Location	*Where does it hurt? Can you point it out? Is it localized or diffuse?* Hint: somatic pain is more localized, whereas visceral pain is diffuse and often described as vague.
Intensity	*On a scale from 0–10, where 0 is no pain and 10 the worst pain you have felt in your life, how would you rate your pain in general? What has been the worst you have experienced? On the same scale, how low does it go after taking pain medication, if any?*
Quality	*How would you best describe your pain?* Hint: burning, shooting pain most often describes neuropathic pain origin, whereas sharp or aching best describes somatic pain.
Timing	*When does it hurt the most? Do you wake up in the middle of the night in pain?* Hint: pain that increases or intensifies at certain times of the day generally indicates that the medication dosage is inadequate.
Duration	*Is the pain constant or intermittent?* Hint: constant pain may be secondary to musculoskeletal involvement. Intermittent pain may be secondary to visceral involvement and is often referred as "colicky."
Radiation	*Does it travel to any other part of your body?* Hint: pain that follows a dermatomal distribution may be secondary to radiculopathy.
Factors that relieve or provoke pain	*Does it get worse with movement? What does make the pain go away? Does it get better if you lay down? Does light touch elicit the pain?* Hint: pain that increases with movement may signify bony involvement of that limb. Pain that intensifies in the recumbent position may mean involvement of the spine. Pain that worsens with a light touch (allodynia) is consistent with neuropathic pain.

2. Assessment of concurrent distressing symptoms: assessment of concomitant distressful symptoms and symptoms caused by other comorbidities. Validated symptom assessment tools such as Edmonton Symptom Assessment Scale can be used.[22,23]
3. Functional status: assessment of activities of daily living and instrumental activities of daily living. Performance status (Karnofsky performance scale[24] or Eastern Cooperative Oncology Group[25] scale scores).
4. Spiritual assessment for spiritual distress/spiritual pain.
5. Assessing for caregiver's distress and/or sociocultural, including financial, issues.

Goal Setting

The therapeutic approach to a patient with serious illness is guided by several goals that are dynamic and evolve over time. The goals are influenced by attitudes and expectations of the patients and their families. Immediate and long-term goals for pain management must be assessed and documented. A therapeutic approach focused on pain only may not suffice for a patient whose suffering is caused by many other reasons. Clinicians who prescribe opioid analgesics for the treatment of chronic pain must understand the regulations and laws that govern the use of controlled prescription drugs and assess and stratify risk in every case and structure treatment plan that is consistent with the perceived risk of abuse and addiction.

Therapeutic Plan

Approach to pain management in patients with advanced illness requires multidimensional assessment and management. It includes pharmacologic and nonpharmacologic interventions customized to the patient's progressive disease and comorbidities. This article focuses on pharmacotherapy of pain.

In recognizing the need for improved pain management worldwide, the World Health Organization (WHO) instituted a 3-step analgesic ladder (**Fig. 1**) as a basis for pain management.[26] This stepwise guide to pain control serves as a basis for its management. Around-the-clock dosing, using adjuvant treatments noninvasive routes of administration provide good pain control for 80% of patients with chronic pain. The types of pain medications should be changed according to the severity of the pain, using the following approach as a guide to maximize pain relief.[12] Numerous studies have shown that when the WHO treatment guidelines are followed, 90% of patients have pain relief.[27] For patients with mild to severe cancer-associated pain, strong opioids can be initiated at low doses as initial step.[28,29]

PHARMACOLOGIC MANAGEMENT OF CHRONIC PAIN
Nonsteroidal Antiinflammatory Drugs

Nonsteroidal antiinflammatory drugs (NSAIDs) prevent formation of prostanoids from arachidonic acid. Prostanoids are subclass of eicosanoids consisting of the prostaglandins (mediators of inflammation), the thromboxanes (mediators of vasoconstriction), and prostacyclins. The synthesis of prostaglandins from arachidonic acid is controlled by 2 separate cyclooxygenase enzymes (COX-1 and COX-2). Nonselective NSAIDs inhibit both COX-1 and COX-2, a nonselective inhibition that results in not only an antiinflammatory response but also a reduced gastrointestinal cytoprotection. COX-2 inhibitors were designed to selectively inhibit only this enzyme, thus maintaining an antiinflammatory response with low risk of side effects that occur with nonselective inhibitors of COX enzymes.[30]

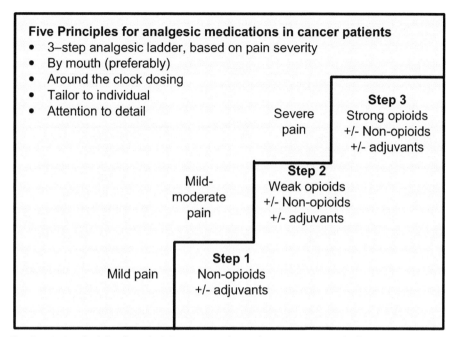

Five Principles for analgesic medications in cancer patients
- 3–step analgesic ladder, based on pain severity
- By mouth (preferably)
- Around the clock dosing
- Tailor to individual
- Attention to detail

Severe pain
Step 3
Strong opioids
+/- Non-opioids
+/- adjuvants

Mild-moderate pain
Step 2
Weak opioids
+/- Non-opioids
+/- adjuvants

Mild pain
Step 1
Non-opioids
+/- adjuvants

Fig. 1. WHO principles for administering analgesic for cancer pain relief.

NSAIDs play a key role in the first step of the management of pain.[31] The NSAIDs include acetaminophen, salicylates (aspirin, salsalate), propionic acid derivatives such as ibuprofen, and acetic acid derivatives (indomethacin, ketorolac) (**Table 2**). In patients with cancer, the use of NSAIDs may delay the development of tolerance and allow the use of a lower dose of opioids with fewer side effects. Because there is no clearly superior NSAID, the choice should be based on pain intensity and underlying disease.[32] All NSAIDs should be avoided in patients with asthma or with known allergy to aspirin. High-risk patients should be started on celecoxib to minimize gastrointestinal ulcers and bleeding. Patients with thrombocytopenia or coagulation disorders can receive celecoxib, choline magnesium salicylate, or salsalate without increased risk for bleeding.

Acetaminophen

The analgesic mechanisms underlying the benefit of acetaminophen are poorly understood but may involve inhibition of prostaglandin formation in the central nervous system, as well as other mechanisms. In contrast to NSAIDs, acetaminophen does not have antiinflammatory properties.[33] Acetaminophen can be used alone or in combination with other opioids (codeine, hydrocodone, oxycodone). When used in combination with opioids, it may have opioid sparing effect.[34]

Opioid Analgesics

A fundamental understanding of the basic and clinical pharmacology of opioids is required to manage both favorable and adverse opioid effects. Long-term opioid therapy is not endorsed for other chronic pain conditions comparable to that achieved for cancer-associated pain. An opioid trial might be considered for any patient with severe chronic pain, but decision to continue requires favorable prediction that benefits

Table 2
Commonly prescribed nonsteroidal antiinflammatory drugs in adults

Medication	Dose	Maximal Dose	Dose Interval	Comments
Acetaminophen[33]	650–1000 mg	Maximal total daily dose: 4 g/d	Q4–6 h	Effective for noninflammatory pain; may be opioid sparing.
Naproxen	Initial dose: 500 mg, then 250 mg	1500 mg	Q6–8 h	Suspension formulation available.
Ibuprofen	400–600 mg	3200 mg	Q6–8 h	Suspension formulation available.
Diclofenac	50 mg	150 mg	Q8–12 h	Diclofenac is also available as a topical patch, solution, and gel.
Meloxicam	7.5–15 mg	15 mg	QD	Long duration of effect; slow onset. Relatively COX-2 selective and minimal effect on platelet function at lower total daily dose of 7.5 mg.
Celecoxib	100–200 mg	200 mg	Q12–24 h	Relative reduction in GI toxicity compared with nonselective NSAIDs.[48] No effect on platelet function.

Abbreviation: GI, gastrointestinal tract.
Data from Davis MP, Dalal S, Goforth H, et al, editors. In: Pain assessment and management. Chicago, IL: AAHPM; 2017. p. 82-85.

will exceed risks. The general approach to chronic opioid therapy and painful crisis is summarized in **Fig. 2** and discussed later.

Opioids are the mainstay for the treatment of moderate to severe pain in patients with advanced illness. Opioid drugs mimic and amplify the actions of endogenous opioid neurotransmitters and the receptors. There are 3 primary opioid receptor types that mediate analgesia: $\mu, \kappa,$ and δ. Drugs that bind to opioid receptors are classified as agonists and antagonists. Most opioids are like the prototype morphine and called as full μ-agonists. Agonist antagonist drugs such as buprenorphine are also called as partial agonist. Less potent opioids such as codeine and hydrocodone are used initially unless patient is in severe pain. These medications are frequently combined with acetaminophen or aspirin and are prescribed as 1 to 2 tablets every 4 hours as needed for pain. Once these opioids are no longer effective, consideration must be given to changing to a stronger opioid as part of the third step in the WHO ladder.[12] Opioids can be obtained in an immediate release (IR) form and a sustained-release (SR) form with dosing of every 8, 12, or 24 hours. Sustained-release preparations cannot be given via gastrostomy tube because of problems with uncontrolled and variable release if pills are crushed or cut.

Opioids are associated with many side effects and complications. Common side effects include sedation, constipation, nausea, and vomiting. Appropriate identification and treatment of the adverse effects are required clinical skills to improve patient's adherence and decrease complications[35] (**Table 3**).

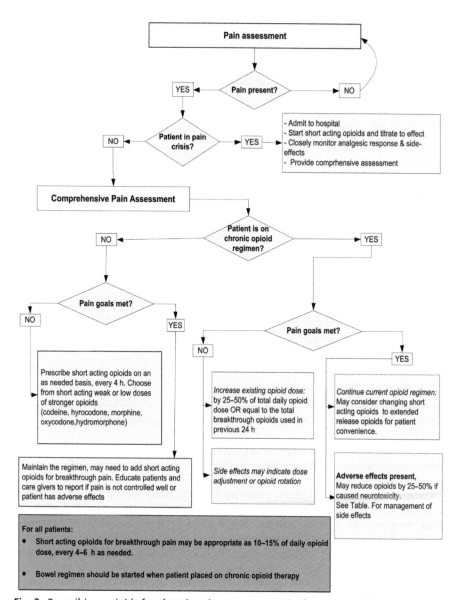

Fig. 2. Prescribing opioids for chronic pain management in the seriously ill.

Morphine is the primary opioid used in the United States for treatment of patients with severe pain. Morphine is primarily metabolized in the liver and its metabolites are excreted renally. Two active metabolites have been extensively studied, morphine-6-glucuronide (M6G) and morphine-3-glucuronide (M3G). Both M3G and M6G cross the blood-brain barrier. M6G seems to contribute to analgesia. In contrast, M3G may be associated with toxic effects, especially in patients with renal failure.[36–38] Morphine is available in once-daily and twice-daily SR oral formulations, IR tablets, oral solutions or elixirs, suppositories, and injectable solutions.

Table 3	
Common opioid side effects	
Side Effect	**Management Strategies**
Nausea/vomiting	Initiate antiemetic medication, explore other causes of nausea. Try to reduce opioid dose if pain is well controlled. Consider opioid rotation if not resolved.
Opioid-induced constipation	Start laxative in all patients on opioids. Rule out fecal impaction. Stimulant laxatives (eg, senna, lactulose, polyethylene glycol). Enemas. Methylnaltrexone, naloxegol.
Neurotoxicity	Opioid rotation/dose reduction. Discontinue other drugs causing CNS depression. Maintain hydration. Explore and treat other causes such as infection, end-organ dysfunction, hypercalcemia, and hyponatremia. Haldol 1–2 mg IV/SubQ q4 h prn.
Respiratory depression	Monitor all opioid-naïve patients closely during first 24 h of initiation of strong opioids. Stop opioid and provide supplemental oxygen. Administer naloxone, 0.4 mg, diluted in 10 mL saline, 1 mL IV push repeat every 1–2 min until patient is awake and respiratory rate improves.
Pruritus	Less likely to occur with fentanyl and oxymorphone. Trial of diphenhydramine or hydroxyzine. Serotonin uptake inhibitors (eg, paroxetine). Gabapentin. Low-dose naloxone. Opioid rotation.

Abbreviations: CNS, central nervous system; IV, intravenous, SubQ, subcutaneous.

Oxycodone and hydromorphone are semisynthetic opioid analgesics that are considered to be comparable to morphine in its pharmacologic actions. Both are available in IR and SR tablets.

As morphine, fentanyl is a strong μ agonist. Fentanyl is highly lipophilic and available as transdermal long-acting opioid. It has no active metabolites and is less likely to cause neurotoxicity. The fentanyl patch is applied once every 3 days and delivers 12, 25, 37.5, 50, 75, 100 μg/h of fentanyl.

Meperidine is not recommended for chronic opioid therapy due to its highly neurotoxic metabolite.

Methadone has variable and unpredictable half-life (15–60 hours) that can make it difficult to be managed by clinicians without experience. Its half-life does not match with observed duration for analgesic effect (6–12 hours). Methadone can cause QT interval prolongation when used at higher doses and combined with other drugs causing QT prolongation. Methadone is recommended for use in late stages after failure of other opioid therapy and only by clinicians with specific training in the risks and uses.[39]

Relative Analgesic Potency

The concept of relative analgesic potency has important implications for the clinical use of opioids. Numerous controlled trials have been done to calculate relative potencies between different opioids given by different routes. These studies have allowed the creation of equianalgesic dose table (**Table 4**). The data it contains were developed from studies in selected populations and cannot be generalized.

Table 4
Opioid equianalgesic table: dosage and duration of action based on single-dose studies

Drug		Equianalgesic Doses (mg)	Duration of Action (h)
Morphine	IV/IM/subQ	10	4–6
	Oral ER	30	8–12
	Oral IR	30	4
	Oral CR[a]	30	8–12
	Oral SR[b]	30	12–24
	Rectal	10	4–24[d,e,f]
Codeine	IM/SQ	N/A	N/A
	Oral	200	4–6
Fentanyl	IV	0.1	1–2
	Oral transmucosal	0.2–0.4	<1
	Transdermal	12.5 mcg/h	48–72
Hydrocodone	Oral	30	4–6
	Oral ER[c]	30	24
Hydromorphone	IM/subQ	1.5–2	4–5
	Rectal	–	6–8
	Oral	7.5	4–6
Methadone	IM/subQ	2–2.5	3–8
	Oral	2.5–15[g]	4–10[h]
Oxycodone	Oral	20	4–6
	Oral CR	20	8–12
Oxymorphone	IM/subQ	1–1.5	4–5
	Oral	10	4–6
Oxycodone	Oral SR	10	8–12
	Rectal	10	4–6
Tapentadol	Oral	50–75	3–7
Tramadol	Oral	50–75	3–7
Agonists-Antagonists	Oral	1	6–8
Buprenorphine	Transdermal	5–10 mcg/h	4–7 d

Abbreviations: CR, controlled release; ER, extended release; SR, sustained release.
  [a] MS Contin(R), Oramorph SR(R).
  [b] Kadian(R) or Avinza(R).
  [c] Zohydro(R) ER.
  [d] IR suppositories have slightly longer durations than oral morphine; CR suppositories may have 12- or 24-hour durations.
  [e] Not recommended in adults for severe pain; not recommended in children.
  [f] No specific recommendations regarding conversion from other oral or parenteral opioids to Embeda. Generally, the safest approach is to give half estimated 24-hour morphine dose and supplement with immediate release morphine for breakthrough pain.
  [g] Dose ratio may increase as the dose of morphine increases.
  [h] Increases with repeated dosing.
Data from Kane CM, Mulvey MR, Wright S, et al. Opioids combined with antidepressants or antiepileptic drugs for cancer pain: Systematic review and meta-analysis. Palliat Med. 2018;32(1):276.

These tables can be used as starting point for starting and switching opioids and routes for administration.[40]

Long-term use of opioids is associated with physical dependence and tolerance. These 2 physiologic processes have nothing to do with addiction, which is psychological. Tolerance is defined as a physiologic phenomenon of progressive decline in the potency of an opioid with continued use, manifested by the requirement of increasing opioid dose to achieve the same therapeutic effect.[41] Tolerance may occur in any pa-tient taking narcotics for more than 1 or 2 weeks and increased doses can continue to provide adequate analgesia with the risk of increase side effects thus limiting its use. Rotating opioids reduces tolerance. Switching from one opioid to another can be accomplished with minimum periods of inadequate analgesia by using a standard equianalgesic table for conversion. When doing opioid rotation, a 25% to 50% dose reduction can be done in order to account for incomplete cross-tolerance.

Dependence is a physiologic process that is independent of tolerance and charac-terized by withdrawal symptoms on abrupt discontinuation or reduction of a chroni-cally administered drug.

Risk Assessment

It is important to assess risk in every patient, even those who are receiving long-term opioid therapy for chronic pain associated with serious illness. The easiest approach to risk assessment is based on information obtained from the history and ancillary sources. It is widely accepted that the risk of abuse or addiction is increased in those with (1) history of drug abuse, (2) major psychiatric disorder, (3) family history of drug abuse, and (4) current dysfunctional and chaotic living environment. Thorough risk assessment and management strategies may reduce the likelihood of problems.[42,43]

CLINICAL PRACTICE POINTS: PRESCRIBING OPIOIDS

- For opioid-naïve patient, start with the lowest dose of IR release and prescribe breakthrough opioid every 4 hours as needed.
- Reassess pain in 3 to 4 days; if patient requiring more than 4 to 6 doses a day, start a long-acting opioid by calculating the 24-hour opioid requirements.
- All patients should have access to breakthrough medication, because up to two-thirds of patients with well-controlled chronic cancer pain have transitory break-through pain.[44] Titrating the opioid can be accomplished either by adding the to-tal amount of breakthrough medication to the long-acting preparation or by increasing the dose by 25% to 50% from the previous day depending on the severity of the patient's pain.[45]
- Reassess pain in 2 to 4 weeks. Frequent pain reassessment is crucial to monitor for desired analgesic effect and/or side effects. Always prescribe a bowel regimen.

Adjuvant Analgesics

Even though opioids are the main analgesic regimen for moderate to severe pain in the terminally ill, adjuvant medications can also be used as the first step or in conjunction with opioids. Adjuvants can be categorized based on how they are used in clinical practice (**Table 5**).

Drugs used for neuropathic pain
The medication selection depends on concomitant symptoms:

- For patients who are experiencing depressive mood, first-line therapy should be an antidepressant. Preferred options include a serotonin-norepinephrine reup-take inhibitor such as duloxetine or a secondary tricyclic drug such as nortripty-line and desipramine (tertiary amines such as amitriptyline, imipramine, doxepin, and clomipramine should be avoided in this patient population, given higher inci-dence of anticholinergic effects, especially sedation).

Table 5
Adjuvants for neuropathic pain

Medication	Dose	Comments
Anticonvulsants		
Gabapentin	900–3600 mg/d	Starting dose of 300 mg/d (1 dose at bedtime or in 3 divided doses). Increase by 100 mg every 3 d
Pregabalin	150–300 mg twice daily	Starting dose of 50–75 mg per day Increase to 100–150 mg/d in 2 divided doses after a few days
Alpha-2 adrenergic agonists		
Tizanidine	16 mg/d	Initial: 2 mg up to 3 times daily May increase based on response and tolerability in 2–4 mg increments per dose
Antidepressants		
Duloxetine	60 mg PO per day	Starting dose of 30 mg/d Increase to 60 mg PO per day in 1 wk Requires 2–4 wk taper if discontinued Avoid use if CrCl <30 mL/min or ESRD
Desipramine	300 mg/d (night time)	Starting dose: 10–25 mg at night Increase slowly at 5–7 d intervals Usual effective antidepressant dose is between 50 and 150 mg/d If more than 100 mg/d, an electrocardiogram should be checked for QTc interval monitoring
Nortriptyline	80 mg/d (divided in 1 to 2 doses)	Staring dose: 20 mg/d
Gaba agonists		
Baclofen	5 mg 3 times a day Increase by 5 mg every third day.	Target dose: 40–80 mg in 24 h
Adjuvants for Bone Pain		
Osteoclast inhibitors		
Pamidronate	60–90 mg IV over 2 h every 3–4 wk	Caution in renal insufficiency
Alendronic acid	4–8 mg IV over 15 min every 4 wk	Caution in renal insufficiency
Denosumab	120 mg subQ every 4 wk	

(continued on next page)

Table 5 (continued)		
Medication	**Dose**	**Comments**
Radiopharmaceuticals		
Strontium-89, samarium-153, radium-223		Induces significant cytopenias Contraindicated in hypercalcemia
Glucocorticoids		
Dexamethasone	4–6 mg PO daily or twice daily (may give loading dose of 10–20 mg if pain is severe)	Taper if given for more than 7 d

Abbreviations: ESRD, end-stage renal disease; IV, intravenous; SubQ, subcutaneous.
Data from Refs.[49–53]

- For patients who are not experiencing depressive mood, first-line therapy should be gabapentin or pregabalin.
- For refractory cases, second-line therapy includes other anticonvulsants (levetiracetam, carbamazepine, oxcarbazepine, valproate, phenytoin, topiramate, lamotrigine, or lacosamide) and alpha-2 adrenergic agonists (tizanidine).

Drugs used for bone pain
Bone pain secondary to tumor expansion and inflammation is a common symptom of some cancers. Pain can be secondary to a single or multiple bone lesions.

- For multifocal bone pain, use NSAIDs, if not contraindicated, and opioids, with or without adjuvant analgesics. Adjuvant analgesics in this setting include osteoclast inhibitors (bisphosphonates, calcitonin, denosumab) and glucocorticoids (dexamethasone is usually preferred for the management of cancer-related pain, given its long half-life and relatively low mineralocorticoid effects), and for refractory cases, bone-seeking radiopharmaceuticals (strontium chloride-89, samarium-153, rhenium-188) can be considered. These treatments may provide pain relief in up to 80% of patients with diffuse metastasis from prostate or breast cancer.[46]
- For single bone lesion, NSAID, if not contraindicated, and opioids, with radiation therapy or/and intervention such as kyphoplasty or surgery.

Topical Coanalgesics

Topical analgesics can be helpful in selected cases and have limited utility in cancer pain.

- Topical lidocaine: lidocaine can be applied as a gel, cream, or patch, also available in combination with prilocaine. Topical lidocaine patch (5%) was shown to be effective in patients with neuropathic pain.[47] Lidocaine systemic absorption is minimal with no systemic side effects. As many as 3 patches can be used concurrently. The patch should not be used over broken skin.
- Capsaicin: capsaicin is a peptide that depletes substance P, which is one of the most important neurotransmitters for pain transmission from peripheral nerves to spinal cord. It has been approved by Food and Drug Administration for arthritis, postsurgical neuropathic pain, and postherpetic neuralgia.

CLINICAL PRACTICE POINTS

- Most patients with serious illness and chronic pain require treatment with opioids. The clinicians should be aware of comprehensive risk assessment and management options. Comprehensive pain assessment remains as the foundation of effective pain management.
- Effective pain management requires customized approach to the type and intensity of pain.
- Be aware of pitfalls of polypharmacy.
- Give lower initial doses of centrally acting medications and opioids in older persons and titrate slowly, involve caregivers' home nursing services to monitor effectiveness of the regimen and side effects.

REFERENCES

1. Caraceni A, Portenoy RK. An international survey of cancer pain characteristics and syndromes. IASP task force on cancer pain. International Association for the Study of Pain. Pain 1999;82:263–74.
2. Clark D. 'Total pain', disciplinary power and the body in the work of Cicely Saunders, 1958-1967. Soc Sci Med 1999;49(6):727–36.
3. Tanaka K, Akechi T, Okuyama T, et al. Impact of Dyspnea, pain and fatigue on daily life activities in ambulatory patients with advanced lung cancer. J Pain Symptom Manage 2002;23:417–23.
4. Webster LR, Beth Dove. Avoiding opioid abuse while managing pain. A guide for practitioners. North Branch, MN: Sunrise River Press; 2007.
5. Broglio K, Portenoy R. Pain assessment and pain management in the last weeks of life. UpToDate. Available at: https://www.uptodate.com/contents/pain-assessment-and-management-in-the-last-weeks-of-life/print. Last Accessed September 25, 2018.
6. Morrison RS, Dietrich J, Meier DE. America's Care of serious illness: a state by state report card on access to palliative care in our nation's hospitals. New York: Center to Advance Palliative Care; 2015. Available at: https://central.capc.org. Accessed September 15, 2018.
7. Caraceni A, Brunelli C, Martini C, et al. Cancer pain assessment in clinical trials. A review of the literature (1999e2002). J Pain Symptom Manage 2005;29(5):507–19.
8. Cleeland CS, Gonin R, Hatfield AK, et al. Pain and its treatment in outpatients with metastatic can- cer. N Engl J Med 1994;330(9):592–6.
9. International Association for the Study of Pain: classification of chronic pain Descriptions of chronic pain syndromes and definitions of pain terms. Prepared by the International Association for the Study of Pain, Subcommittee on Taxonomy. Pain 1986;(Suppl):S1–226.
10. Chou R, Fanciullo GJ, Fine PG, et al. Clinical guidelines for the use of chronic opioid therapy in chronic noncancer pain. J Pain 2009;10(2):113–30.
11. Fine PG. Long-term consequences of chronic pain: mounting evidence for pain as a neurological disease and parallels with other chronic disease states. Pain Med 2011;12(7):996–1004.
12. Perron V, Schonwetter RS. Assessment and management of pain in palliative care patients. Cancer Control 2001;8(1):15–24.
13. Turk DC, Monarch ES, Williams AD. Cancer patients in pain: considerations for assessing the whole person. Hematol Oncol Clin North Am 2002;16(3):511–25.
14. Chang HM. Cancer pain management. Med Clin North Am 1999;83:711–36.

15. Baron R, Binder A, Wasner G. Neuropathic pain: diagnosis, pathophysiology mechanisms, and treatment. Lancet Neurol 2010;9(8):807–19.
16. Bouhassira D, Attal N. Translational neuropathic pain research: a clinical perspective. Neuroscience 2016;338:27–35.
17. Hjermstad MJ, Fainsinger R, Kaasa S, European Palliative Care Research Collaborative (EPCRC). Assessment and classification of cancer pain. Curr Opin Support Palliat Care 2009;3:24–30.
18. Herr K, Bjoro K, Decker S. Tools for assessment of pain in nonverbal older adults with dementia: a state of the science review. J Pain Symptom Manage 2006; 31(2):170–92.
19. Portenoy R, Conn M. Cancer pain syndromes. In: Bruera E, Portenoy R, editors. Cancer pain assessment and management, vol. 1, 1st edition. New York: Cambridge University Press; 2003. p. 89–108.
20. Mehta A, Chan LS. Understanding of the concept of "Total pain": a prerequisite for pain control. J Hosp Palliat Nurs 2008;10(1):26–32.
21. Bruera E, Higginson I, Von Gunten C, et al. Textbook of palliative medicine and supportive care. Boca Raton, FL: CRC Press; 2015.
22. Bruera E, Kuehn N, Miller MJ, et al. The Edmonton Symtom Assessment System (ESAS): a simple method for the assessment of palliative care patients. J Palliat Care 1991;7(2):6–9.
23. Fainsinger RL, Nekolaichuk CL, Lawlor PG, et al. A multicenter study of the revised Edmonton Staging System for classifying cancer pain in advanced cancer patients. J Pain Symptom Manage 2005;29(3):224–37.
24. Schag CC, Heinrich RL, Ganz PA. Karnofsky performance status revisited: reliability, validity, and guidelines. J Clin Oncol 1984;2:187–93.
25. Oken M, Creech R, Tormey D, et al. Toxicity and response criteria of the Eastern Cooperative Oncology Group. Am J Clin Oncol 1982;5:649–55.
26. World Health Organization. Cancer pain relief and palliative care: report of a WHO Expert Committee. Geneva (Switzerland): WHO; 1990. p. 804. Technical report series, 0512-3054.
27. Pharo GH, Zhou L. Pharmacologic management of cancer pain. J Am Osteopath Assoc 2005;105(11 Suppl 5):S21–8.
28. Mercadante S, Porzio G, Ferrera P, et al. Low morphine doses in opioid –naïve cancer patients with pain. J Pain Symptom Manage 2006;31(3):242–7.
29. Marinangeli F, Ciccizzi A, Leonardis M, et al. Use of strong opioids in advanced cancer pain: a randomized trial. J Pain Symptom Manage 2004;27(5):409–16.
30. Stockler M, Vardy J, Pillai A, et al. Acetaminophen (paracetomal) improves pain and well-being in people with advanced cancer already receiving a strong opioid regimen: a randomized, double-blind, placebo-controlled crossover trial. J Clin Oncol 2004;22:3389–94.
31. Silvestri GA, Sherman C, Williams T, et al. Caring for the dying patient with lung cancer. Chest 2002;122:1028–36.
32. Mercadante S. The use of anti-inflammatory drugs in cancer pain. Cancer Treat Rev 2001;27(1):51–61.
33. Twycross R, Pace V, Mihalyo M, et al. Acetaminophen (paracetamol). J Pain Symptom Manage 2013;46(5):747–55.
34. McNicol E, Strassels SA, Goudas L, et al. NSAIDs or paracetamol, alone or combined with opioids for cancer pain. Cochrane Database Syst Rev 2005;(1):CD005180.
35. Benyamin R, Trescot AM, Datta S, et al. Opioid complications and side effects. Pain Physician 2008;11:S105–20.

36. Faura CC, Moore RA, Horga JF, et al. Morphine and morphine-6-glucuronide plasma concentrations and effect in cancer pain. J Pain Symptom Manage 1996;11(2):95.
37. Tiseo PJ, Thaler HT, Lapin J, et al. Morphine-6-glucuronide concentrations and opioid-related side effects: a survey in cancer patients. Pain 1995;61(1):47.
38. D'Honneur G, Gilton A, Sandouk P, et al. Plasma and cerebrospinal fluid concentrations of morphine and morphine glucuronides after oral morphine. The influence of renal failure. Anesthesiology 1994;81(1):87.
39. Manchikanti L, Abdi S, Atluri S, et al. American Society of Interventional Pain Physicians (ASIPP) guidelines for responsible opioid prescribing in chronic non-cancer pain: part 2–guidance. Pain Physician 2012;15(3 Suppl):S67–116.
40. Shaheen PE, Walsh D, Lasheen W, et al. Opioid equianalgesic tables: are they all equally dangerous? J Pain Symptom Manage 2009;38(3):409–17.
41. Wootton M. Morphine is not the only analgesic in palliative care: literature review. J Adv Nurs 2004;45:527–32.
42. Gourlay D, Heit H, Almahrezi A. Universal precautions in pain medicine: a rational approach to treatment of chronic pain. Pain Med 2005;6:107–12.
43. Ballantyne JC, LaForge KS. Opioid dependence and addiction during opioid treatment of chronic pain. Pain 2007;129:235–55.
44. Bruera E, Neumann CM. Role of methadone in the management of pain in cancer patients. Oncology 1999;13:1275–82.
45. Portenoy RK, Lesage P. Management of cancer pain. Lancet 1999;353:1695–700.
46. Abrahm JL. A physician's guide to pain and symptom management in cancer patients. 2nd edition. In: Wehmueller J, editor. Baltimore, MD: The John Hopkins University Press; 2005. p. 211–3.
47. Galer BS, Jensen MP, Ma T, et al. The lidocaine patch 5% effectively treats all neuropathic pain qualities: results of a randomized, double-blind, vehicle controlled,3-week efficacy study with use of the neuropathic pain scale. Clin J Pain 2002;18:297–301.
48. Castellsague J, Riera-Guardia N, Calingaert B, et al. Individual NSAIDs and upper gastrointestinal complications: a systematic review. Drug Saf 2012;35:1127.
49. Kane CM, Mulvey MR, Wright S, et al. Opioids combined with antidepressants or antiepileptic drugs for cancer pain: systematic review and meta-analysis. Palliat Med 2018;32(1):276.
50. Saarto T, Wiffen PJ. Antidepressants for neuropathic pain. Cochrane Database Syst Rev 2007;(4):CD005454.
51. Jongen JL, Huijsman ML, Jessurun J, et al. The evidence for pharmacologic treatment of neuropathic cancer pain: beneficial and adverse effects. J Pain Symptom Manage 2013;46(4):581–90.e1.
52. Hendriks LE, Hermans BC, van den Beuken-van Everdingen MH, et al. Effect of bisphosphonates, denosumab, and radioisotopes on bone pain and quality of life in patients with non-small cell lung cancer and bone metastases: a systematic review. J Thorac Oncol 2016;11(2):155.
53. Abraham J. Pharmacologic management of cancer pain. In: A physician's guide to pain and symptom management in cancer patients. Baltimore (MD): Johns Hopkins University Press; 2005. p. 261–2.

Nonpain Symptom Management

Olumuyiwa O. Adeboye, MBBS, MBA

KEYWORDS

- Anorexia • Constipation • Nausea and vomiting

KEY POINTS

- This article provides an overview of the management of three very common nonpain symptoms that are often unrecognized in the setting of advanced illness, ad typically encountered by primary care clinicians, specifically, anorexia, constipation and nausea.
- Anorexia is a common and frequently concerning symptom among patients with advanced illnesses and its presence usually indicates disease progression.
- Constipation, a subjective symptom for most patients with advanced illness, can lead to serious complications if left unmanaged and can be easily assessed and treated.
- Understanding the pathways involved in nausea and vomiting can help identify the cause and is very important in pharmacologic management.

Primary care clinicians, because of their relationships with patients with advanced/serious illnesses, are key in helping manage the many common symptoms (**Fig. 1**) other than pain that affect the quality of life of these patients. Basic symptom management, which can be a burden for most clinicians for several reasons, when done well can promote stronger clinician-patient relationships and helps reduce fragmentation of care.[1] A familiarity with the patient's preferences and goals of care and incorporating these into an individualized care plan can also help achieve the so-called triple aim of health care reform.[2]

This article provides an overview of the management of common nonpain symptoms in the setting of advanced illness, encountered by primary care clinicians; specifically, anorexia, constipation, nausea, and vomiting.

For the purposes of this article, an advanced illness is defined as "occurring when one or more conditions become serious enough that general health and functioning decline, and treatments begin to lose their impact. This is a process that continues to the end of life."[3]

Disclosure: The author has nothing to disclose.
Palliative Care, Ascension Wisconsin, Ascension St. Elizabeth Hospital Campus, 1611 South Madison Street, Office 1A005, Appleton, WI 54915, USA
E-mail address: olumuyiwa.adeboye@ascension.org

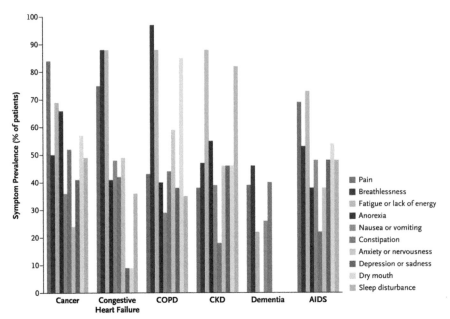

Fig. 1. Symptom prevalence in advanced illnesses. AIDS, acquired immunodeficiency syndrome; CKD, chronic kidney disease; COPD, chronic obstructive pulmonary disease. (*From* Kelley AS, Morrison RS. Palliative care for the seriously ill. N Engl J Med 2015;373:749; with permission.)

ANOREXIA

Meaning without appetite or desire to eat,[4] anorexia is a common symptom among patients with advanced illnesses. It is associated with cachexia, frequently unrecognized and untreated, and is often a great concern to patients and their families. Its presence usually indicates disease progression.

Prevalence

Anorexia has been reported in 50% of patients with advanced disease at the time of diagnosis, and in as many as 85% of patients with advanced cancer.[5,6] It typically ends up causing a reduction in caloric intake, malnutrition, and weight loss and is common in many disease entities. In adults with chronic kidney disease, 30% to 40% on maintenance hemodialysis reported anorexia, which was associated with increased rates of hospitalization, poor quality of life, and increased mortality.[7] Inadequate caloric intake with its attendant malnutrition is common in most patients with heart failure[8] and in about 20% to 40% of outpatients with chronic obstructive pulmonary disease, going to as high as 70% when admitted with respiratory failure.[9]

Pathophysiology and Cause

Adequate caloric intake depends on multiple factors, including the palatability of food, which is controlled by the cranial nerves (the olfactory, glossopharyngeal, and facial), and the feeling of satiety, which is mediated by the autonomic sensory nerves innervating the proximal gastrointestinal (GI) tract and contained in the afferent arm of the vagus nerve. Nutritional intake is coordinated by the brain, primarily in the hypothalamic nuclei, which integrates signals from cognitive, visual, and sensory stimuli as well as activity of the GI tract. Signaling molecules, including hormones and neurotransmitters, that exert a stimulating or positive effect on appetite are glucocorticoids, dopamine, ghrelin, orexin A and B, endocannabinoids, and neuropeptide Y. Alpha-melanocyte–stimulating hormone, serotonin, leptin, tumor necrosis factor alpha, pro-opiomelanocortin, and thyrotropin-releasing hormone exert a negative or inhibiting control of appetite.[10–18]

Apart from the advanced illnesses already mentioned earlier, medications, including amphetamines, antibiotics, opioids[19], antihistamines, digoxin, ranolazine, and antidepressants, are also known culprits of anorexia. Aging, because of decreased energy needs and changes in the sense of taste and smell, may contribute to a loss or lack of appetite.[20]

Assessment

All patients with advanced incurable illnesses need to be assessed for anorexia with a careful history, taking into consideration patients' self-report of appetite and early satiety. This self-report is key, along with questions about taste and/or smell alterations, xerostomia, constipation, nausea with or without vomiting, and depression. Patients may also experience uncontrolled pain or abdominal discomfort from ascites, breathlessness, or hiccups.[21] For practical purposes of symptom assessment in patients with advanced illness, the use of multiple symptom assessment tools, such as the revised Edmonton Symptom Assessment System (rESAS), that can recognize unreported symptoms is encouraged (**Fig. 2**). rESAS is a 9-item numeric symptom rating visual analog scale that can also be modified for other symptoms not included, such as constipation. Other tools used in research settings, but that may be too cumbersome for use in an office practice, are available.

Treatment

Nonpharmacologic interventions that encourage patients to enjoy small frequent meals dense in calories and try to sit at the dinner table with other family members are key first steps. Also, emphasizing quality (ie, taste) rather than quantity, is important, along with counseling patients and families about their underlying disease processes. The use of nutritional supplementation may be of benefit to some. For patients with persistent anorexia, treatment should be designed to eliminate the underlying disease process when possible. In addition, optimizing management of major contributors to anorexia, such as nausea and constipation, may result in significant improvement.[22] When this is not possible, treatment involves drug therapies that interfere with the downregulation of cytokine synthesis and release. In addition, treatment is designed to correct underlying physiologic mechanisms such as gastric dysmotility (decreased GI motility, decreased gastric emptying because of disease progression). Decreased gastric motility also may result from opioid therapy, a side effect of which may be constipation, leading to bloating and the feeling of fullness, which interfere with appetite and food intake. Esophageal reflux, mucositis, and oral candidiasis affect taste; poor dentition or ill-fitting dentures and intractable hiccups affect the ability to eat.[6]

Pharmacologic treatments (**Table 1**) predominantly help with appetite stimulation but do not lead to weight gain.

CONSTIPATION

Constipation is commonly defined as the infrequent or difficult evacuation of feces.[23] Although the typical physician definition is fewer than 3 bowel movements per week,[24] it means different things to different people and, as a result, it is best defined according to the individual patient's experience. After pain and anorexia, it is the third most

Please circle the number that best describes how you feel NOW:

| No pain | 0 1 2 3 4 5 6 7 8 9 10 | Worst possible pain |

| No tiredness | 0 1 2 3 4 5 6 7 8 9 10 | Worst possible tiredness |
(Tiredness=lack of energy)

| No drowsiness | 0 1 2 3 4 5 6 7 8 9 10 | Worst possible drowsiness |
(Drowsiness=feeling sleepy)

| No nausea | 0 1 2 3 4 5 6 7 8 9 10 | Worst possible nausea |

| No lack of appetite | 0 1 2 3 4 5 6 7 8 9 10 | Worst possible lack of appetite |

| No shortness of breath | 0 1 2 3 4 5 6 7 8 9 10 | Worst possible shortness of breath |

| No depression | 0 1 2 3 4 5 6 7 8 9 10 | Worst possible depression |
(Depression=feeling sad)

| No anxiety | 0 1 2 3 4 5 6 7 8 9 10 | Worst possible anxiety |
(Anxiety=feeling nervous)

| Best well-being | 0 1 2 3 4 5 6 7 8 9 10 | Worst possible well-being |
(Well-being=how you feel overall)

| No _____ | 0 1 2 3 4 5 6 7 8 9 10 | Worst possible _____ |
Other problem (for example, constipation)

Patient name: _____
Date: _____
Time: _____

Fig. 2. Edmonton symptom assessment system, revised version. (*From* Watanabe SM, Neko-laichuk C, Beaumont C, et al. A multicenter study comparing two numerical versions of the Edmonton symptom assessment system in palliative care patients. J Pain Symptom Manag 2011;41(2):468; with permission.)

common symptom seen in the palliative medicine patient population.[25] Despite this, it can often go unrecognized, leading to significant morbidity and suffering. Clinical manifestations include abdominal pain, bloating, nausea, vomiting, abdominal distention, loss of appetite, and headache. When left unmanaged, it can lead to complications such as overflow incontinence, tenesmus, fecal impaction, bowel obstruction (obstipation), intestinal perforation, urinary retention or frequency, rectal tearing, rectal fissures, and hemorrhoids.[26]

Table 1
Pharmacologic treatment options for anorexia

Drug	Dose	Comments
Megestrol acetate	Start at 160 mg daily and titrate to maximum dose of 800 mg/d Discontinue if no improvement in appetite within 2 wk	Progesterone derivative Modest beneficial effect on appetite in patients with cancer-related anorexia Limited data in noncancer conditions Avoid in patients with history of deep venous thrombosis, pulmonary embolism, or severe cardiac disease because edema and thromboembolic phenomena are common side effects
Prednisone Dexamethasone	20–40 mg/d 3–4 mg/d	Stimulate appetite in patients with cancer No evidence for use in patients without cancer Short-term use recommended rather than prolonged therapy, which can lead to several side effects, including myopathy
Dronabinol	5–20 mg/d	Benefit limited to increased appetite only, inferior to megestrol Evidence to support use still limited CNS side effects, such as sedation, confusion, and perceptual disturbance limit its use
Metoclopramide	10 mg every 4 h while awake; titrate up to 120 mg/d	5-HT4 receptor agonist Stimulates gastric and duodenal motility decreasing nausea and increasing appetite in patients with gastroparesis
Mirtazapine	7.5–30 mg by mouth at bedtime	Tetracyclic antidepressant that induces weight gain and increases food intake Promising agent for the treatment of cancer-related anorexia with coexisting depression Phase III RCT underway to prove its benefit

Abbreviations: CNS, central nervous system; 5-HT4, 5-hydroxytryptamine type 4; RCT, randomized clinical trial.

Prevalence

In the general North American population, estimates range from 2% to 28%,[27,28] whereas in Solano and colleagues'[29] review, the prevalence of constipation in patients with advanced illness varied. For cancer, it was 23% to 65%, 34% to 35% in acquired immunodeficiency syndrome (AIDS), 38% to 42% in heart disease, 27% to 44% in chronic obstructive pulmonary disease (COPD), and 29% to 70% in renal disease. Also of note, about 50% of patients admitted to palliative care centers report constipation as a problem.[30]

Pathophysiology and Cause

In patients with advanced illness, disturbances in normal bowel habits constipation can be multifactorial with pathologies at multiple levels contributing to altered bowel patterns. **Box 1** highlights various factors contributing to and associated with constipation in advanced illness.

Assessment

A thorough history including details of premorbid bowel habits, the last bowel movement, and associated symptoms, as highlighted earlier, are key in the initial

Box 1
Factors contributing to constipation

Organic factors

Drugs/pharmacologic agents
   Opioid analgesics
   Antihypertensive agents (calcium channel blockers)
   Tricyclic antidepressants
   Iron preparations
   Antiepileptic drugs
   Antiparkinsonian agents
   Barium
   Antacids (calcium and aluminum compounds)
   Antiemetics (seratonin antagonists)
   Antitussives
   Antidiarrheal agents (when used in excess)
   Vinca alkaloids
   Diuretics

Endocrine or metabolic disturbances
   Diabetes mellitus
   Hypothyroidism
   Hypercalcemia
   Porphyria
   Chronic renal insufficiency
   Panhypopituitarism
   Hypokalemia
   Dehydration
   Pregnancy

Neurologic disorders
   Spinal cord injury
   Parkinson disease
   Multiple sclerosis
   Autonomic neuropathy
   Hirschsprung disease
   Chronic intestinal pseudo-obstruction
   Cerebral tumors

Structural abnormalities
   Pelvic tumor mass from colorectal cancer or extraintestinal mass
   Postinflammatory, ischemic, or surgical stenosis from radiation fibrosis
   Myogenic: myotonic dystrophy, dermatomyositis, scleroderma, amyloidosis
   Anorectal: anal fissure, anal strictures, inflammatory bowel disease, proctitis, perianal abscess, hemorrhoids

Functional factors

Dietary
   Low-fiber diet
   Dehydration (from poor fluid intake)
   Poor appetite
   Low amounts of food intake

Environmental
   Lack of privacy
   Comfort
   Assistance with toileting

Others
   Advanced age
   Inactivity
   Decreased mobility

Bed confinement
Depression
Sedation

Data from Wald A. Constipation: advances in diagnosis and treatment. JAMA 2016;315:185–191; and Larkin PJ, Cherny NI, La Carpia D, et al. Diagnosis, assessment and management of constipation in advanced cancer: ESMO clinical practice guidelines. Ann Oncol 2018;29(Supp 4):iv111–iv125.

management. Changes in patterns of stool frequency, consistency, and straining, as well as diet and medications, also need to be inquired about.

A physical examination must include a digital rectal examination looking out for any abnormalities, including masses, fissures and hemorrhoids, assessing the rectal tone and checking for the presence of stool in the rectal vault, and impaction and its consistency. This examination should be avoided in patients with neutropenia and thrombocytopenia unless absolutely necessary.[5]

Diagnostic testing focused on the correctable causes listed earlier can be ordered. The routine use of plain radiographs to assess the degree of constipation has been recommended to be limited to the following clinical scenarios:

1. Concern for bowel obstruction or ischemia
2. Patient with liquid stool most likely from severe constipation
3. Patient with a lifelong history of constipation in whom neurogenic causes of reduced bowel motility are a concern in order to detect megacolon or megarectum
4. Occasionally to monitor the response to laxatives in patients with fecal retention[31]

Treatment

Preventive measures are key and are a major first step in managing constipation. These measures include:

1. Patient education
2. Increasing or maintaining adequate dietary and oral fluid intake
3. Initiating and maintaining a regular bowel regimen with prophylactic laxatives when initiating opioids in patients
4. Encouraging patients to increase mobility if possible
5. Providing a comfortable and private environment for defecation
6. Discontinuing and avoiding medications that can cause constipation

These steps can also be incorporated into the treatment of constipation while also considering pharmacologic interventions.

The common medications used in the treatment of constipation, their mechanisms and onset of action, as well as dosages are listed in **Table 2**.

The optimal laxative regimen is unclear and various options are available and should be individualized based on the patient's condition. There are no randomized trials documenting the superiority of one standard laxative over another, and recommendations are based on consensus opinion and best practice.

NAUSEA AND VOMITING

Nausea is an unpleasant subjective sensation that signals vomiting is imminent, and it may or may not result in vomiting. It is frequently multifactorial and commonly accompanied by other symptoms, including pain, insomnia, anorexia, fatigue, anxiety, and/or depression.[32] Vomiting is the forceful expulsion of gastric contents through the mouth

Table 2
Pharmacologic treatment options for constipation

Laxatives	Mechanism	Recommended Doses	Onset of Action	Comments
Emollients Docusate Mineral oil	Act as detergents and help decrease surface tension	Start 300 mg/d. Maximum 800 mg/d 15–45 mL/d	1–3 d Oral: 6–8 h Rectal: 2–15 min	Ensure adequate fluid intake Ineffectual alone and should only be used in combination with laxatives Lipid pneumonitis with aspiration. Especially in elderly patients
Bulk forming Psyllium Methylcellulose	Natural or synthetic, act by absorbing water in the intestine, increasing stool bulk, thereby promoting peristalsis and reducing transit time	Start 5–7 g/d Start 4–7 g/d	12–72 h 12–72 h	Requires at least 300–500 mL of water ingestion, otherwise impaction may occur
Hyperosmolar agents Lactulose Polyethylene glycol Sorbitol	Undigestible, unabsorbable compounds that remain within and retain water already present in the colon, leading to stool softening	Start: 15–30 mL/d Max: 60 mL/d in 1–2 divided doses 17–34 g/d 30–150 mL (as 70% solution)	24–48 h 48–96 h 24–48 h	Abdominal bloating, colic and flatulence Urticaria Pulmonary edema and hyperglycemia
Stimulants Bisacodyl Senna	Stimulate peristalsis by directly irritating smooth muscle of the intestine, possibly the colonic intramural plexus, alter water and electrolyte secretion, producing net intestinal fluid accumulation and laxation	Start: 5 mg/d Max: 30 mg/d Start: 15 mg/d Max: 70–100 mg/d	6–10 h 6–12 h	Electrolyte and fluid imbalance Nausea, vomiting, melanosis coli
Prokinetic agents Metoclopramide	Promote colonic transit by increasing colonic motor activity	40–120 mg/d 30–80 mg/d	Variable	Extrapyramidal symptoms. Results are not impressive. Consider for refractory constipation. Avoid in cardiac patients

	Mechanism	Dose	Onset	Comments
Opioid antagonists Methylnaltrexone Naloxegol	Mu-receptor antagonist Pegylated derivative of naloxone	38–61 kg: 8 mg 62–114 kg: 12 mg >114 kg: 0.15 mg/kg (round dose up to nearest 0.1 mL of volume) 12.5–25 mg	30–60 min 6–12 h	Only approved for opioid-induced constipation FDA approved for opioid-induced constipation in patients with chronic noncancer pain
Lubiprostone	Selective chloride channel-2 activator	24 μg twice daily	<24 h	FDA approved for opioid-induced constipation in patients with chronic noncancer pain Common adverse effects: nausea, headache and diarrhea
Rectal preparations Sorbitol/lactulose enemas	Hyperosmolar agent	120 mL of sorbitol 25%–30% solution 200–300 mL of lactulose solution mixed with 700 mL of water or saline retained for 30–60 min	0.5–3 h	Also used for hepatic encephalopathy Avoid in patients at risk of bleeding or with rectosigmoid lesions
Saline enemas Glycerin suppository Bisacodyl suppository	Cause water to be drawn into the colon Act by irritating the rectum Acts as a stimulant laxative	Dose varies by the type of saline laxative Single dose 2–3 g/d 10 mg daily	0.5–6 h 0.5–3 h <1 h	Repeated enemas may result in electrolyte disturbances May cause local irritation

Abbreviation: FDA, US Food and Drug Administration.

caused by sustained contraction of abdominal muscles and diaphragm along with the opening of the gastric cardia.

Prevalence

Most studies related to prevalence of nausea and vomiting are in the patients with cancer. Forty percent of patients being treated with chemotherapy or radiation therapy have breakthrough nausea and vomiting and 30% to 60% of those no longer receiving treatments still have nausea and vomiting.[33–39] The review article by Solano and colleagues[29] reported rates of nausea ranging from 17% to 48% in heart disease, 30% to 43% in renal disease, and 43% to 49% in patients with AIDS. A 2009 article by Blinderman and colleagues[40] identified a prevalence of 18% for nausea and 4% for vomiting in patients with advance COPD.

Pathophysiology and Cause

The ability to understand the pathways involved in nausea and vomiting and identify the cause (**Box 2**) is key to pharmacologic management. Vomiting can be triggered by afferent impulses to the vomiting center (VC; located in the medulla) from the chemoreceptor trigger zone (CTZ; located in the area postrema in the floor of the fourth ventricle), GI tract, and cerebral cortex. Vomiting occurs when efferent impulses are sent from the VC to the salivation center, abdominal muscles, respiratory center, and cranial nerves. There are many neurotransmitter receptors in the CTZ, VC, and GI tract. The principal neuroreceptors involved in the emetic response are the serotonin and dopamine receptors (**Fig. 3**).[41] Other neuroreceptors involved include acetylcholine, corticosteroid, histamine, cannabinoid, opioid, and neurokinin-1.[42] Antiemetic drugs are predominantly blocking agents, effective at different receptor sites. Administering the most potent antagonist to the implicated receptor has been shown to be effective in up to 80% to 90% of patients near the end of life.[43]

Assessment

Nausea and vomiting, although separate, are related, can be debilitating, and can cause significant physical and psychological distress to patients and their families.

Box 2
Common causes of nausea and vomiting in advanced illness

Drugs
    Cytotoxic chemotherapy
    Opioids, tramadol
    Nonsteroidal antiinflammatory drugs, aspirin
    Digitalis
    Iron
    Antibiotics
    Theophylline
    Selective serotonin reuptake inhibitors and bupropion
    Anticonvulsants
    Many other drugs
    Medications with anticholinergic side effects
    Polypharmacy

Metabolic/biochemical causes
    Hypercalcemia
    Hyponatremia
    Ketoacidosis
    Liver or renal failure or impairment
    Poisoning, substance abuse
    Infection

GI causes
  Impaired motility: gastroparesis
  Myopathies and neuropathies
  Obstruction: gastric outlet, small bowel, biliary/pancreatic duct
  Inflammation: gastritis, gastroenteritis, hepatitis, cholecystitis, pancreatitis, radiation
  induced
  Severe constipation
  Hyperacidity
  Gastroesophageal reflux disease
  Hepatomegaly, ascites

Neurologic causes
  Increased intracranial pressure: malignancy, hemorrhage, abscess
  Meningeal infiltration/irritation
  Metastases
  Vestibular nerve stimulation: drugs or labyrinthitis
  Pain

Psychological causes
  Anxiety: anticipatory nausea and vomiting
  Depression

Myocardial dysfunction
  Ischemia
  Congestive heart failure

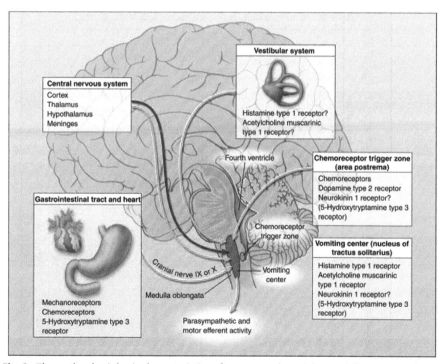

Fig. 3. The pathophysiologic characteristics of nausea and vomiting and the targets of anti-emetic therapies in gastroparesis. (*From* McCallum RW, Sunny JK. Gastroparesis. In: McNally PR, editor. GI/liver secrets plus. Elsevier; 2015. p. 87–94; with permission.)

Table 3
Pharmacologic treatment options for nausea and vomiting

Drug	Receptor and Site	Indications	Dosage and Routes	Side Effects	Notes
Butyrophenones Haloperidol	D_2 CTZ	Opioid-induced and chemical/metabolic nausea	0.5–2 mg every 6–8 h PO, SC, IV	EPS, QTc, somnolence	Side effects unusual at low doses, caution in severe liver impairment, reduce dose by 50% in renal failure
Prokinetic agents Metoclopramide	D_2 CTZ D_2 GIT $5\text{-}HT_4$ GIT (potentiation) $5\text{-}HT_3$ CTZ (at high doses) GIT	Gastric stasis; ileus Chemotherapy	10–20 mg 4 hourly PO, SC, IV NA	EPS, restlessness, drowsiness Colic in GI obstruction	Prolonged half-life in renal failure Superseded by $5\text{-}HT_3$ antagonists
Phenothiazines (including prochlorperazine chlorpromazine)	D_2 CTZ D_2 GIT H_1 VC Ach CNS α_1 Ad GIT	—	Prochlorperazine: 5–10 mg PO, 12.5–25 mg IM, 25 mg PR 6–8 hourly Chlorpromazine: 10–25 mg PO 4 hourly 25–50 mg IM 4–6 hourly	Vary according to spectrum of receptor blockade, QTc	—
Antihistamines Promethazine Diphenhydramine	CTZ H_1 GIT CVS CNS VC vestibular afferents	—	Promethazine: 12–25 mg 8 hourly PO	Dry mouth, blurred vision, sedation, EPS Skin irritation at SC injection sites QTc	Avoid in the elderly
Diphenhydramine	Ach_m brain substance VC	—	—	—	—

	Receptor/site	Indication	Dose	Side effects	Comments
Anticholinergics Hyoscine (scopolamine)	Ach_m VC GIT GIT	Intestinal obstruction; peritoneal irritation; increased ICP; excess secretions	200–400 μg 4–8 hourly SL/SC; 500–1500 μg/72 h transdermal patches; 20 mg PO/SC 6 hourly	Dry mouth, sedation, ileus, urinary retention, blurred vision, occasionally agitation	Useful if NV coexist with colic, illogical to give with prokinetics; Does not cross BB, antisecretory; nonsedative; Poorly absorbed from the GI tract
5-HT₃ antagonists Granisetron Ondansetron Tropisetron Polanesetron Dolasetron	5-HT₃ GIT CTZ (VC)	First-line agents in CINV. Can also be used for abdominal radiotherapy; postoperative NV	Granisetron: 3 mg slowly IV up to 8 hourly; ondansetron: 8 mg PO or slowly IV 8 hourly; tropisetron: 5 mg PO or slowly IV daily; Polanesetron: 250 μg IV daily	Headache in 30%; constipation; diarrhea, dizziness, QTc	Effectiveness increased by combination with dexamethasone; Indicated in NV related to chemotherapy, radiotherapy, or surgery
NK₁ antagonist Aprepitant	NK₁ widespread	Late-onset chemotherapy-related NV	125 mg 1 h before chemotherapy; then 80 mg OD for the next 2 d	Hiccups, asthenia, fatigue, somnolence, anxiety, anorexia, GI upset	Only available PO
Mirtazapine	5-HT₃ GIT	Chemotherapy-related NV	15–45 mg PO qhs	Somnolence at low dose, dry mouth, and increased appetite	FDA approved as an antidepressant (noradrenergic and specific serotonergic); Useful in the elderly and those with insomnia and anorexia; Available as an oral disintegrating tablet

(continued on next page)

Table 3
(continued)

Drug	Receptor and Site	Indications	Dosage and Routes	Side Effects	Notes
Atypical antipsychotic Olanzapine	Multiple D_1, D_2, D_3, D_4 (brain), 5-HT_{2a}, 5-HT_{2c}, 5-HT_3, 5-HT_6, Ach_m, H_1, α_1 Ad	Chemotherapy-induced NV, refractory nausea caused by opioids	10 mg PO once and daily on days 2–4	QT prolongation especially when used with other QT prolonging agents, dystonic reactions	Use with caution with metoclopramide or haloperidol because excessive dopamine blockade can increase EPS Consider 5-mg dose for elderly or oversedated patients Parenteral use contraindicated with concomitant parenteral BZD use
Corticosteroids Dexamethasone	Not well understood, but may antagonize prostaglandin or release endorphins	Additive to other antiemetics in chemotherapy regimens, increased ICP, incomplete mechanical bowel obstruction, postoperatively	8–12 mg PO/IV once or daily	Hyperglycemia, dyspepsia	Use with caution in patients with DM Not recommended with immunotherapy or cellular therapies Consider AM dosing to minimize insomnia

Abbreviations: Ach, Acetylcholine; Ad, Adrenergic; BZD, Benzodiazepine; CVS, Cardiovascular system; CINV, chemotherapy-induced nausea and vomiting; DM, diabetes mellitus; EPS, Extrapyramidal symptoms; GIT, Gastrointestinal tract; 5-HT2 - 5-Hydroxytryptamine receptor subtype 2; IM, intramuscular; ICP, intracranial pressure; IV, intravenous; NA, not available; NK1, Neurokinin receptor subtype; NV, Nausea-Vomiting; OD, once daily; PO, by mouth; PR, Per rectum; qhs, at bedtime; SL, Sublingual; QTc, corrected QT interval; SC, subcutaneous.

A thorough assessment of these symptoms, including a detailed history and thorough physical examination, assists the clinician in understanding the severity and cause. Their management can also provide significant relief and satisfaction to all.[44] Nausea is subjective and, therefore, the clinician must rely on patient report. To record intensity and frequency of nausea, the rESAS can be used, not only at the initial evaluation but also at regular intervals to evaluate the patient's response to treatment.[45] Vomiting may be measured objectively, but the degree of distress is subjective and can only be reported by the individual. Physicians should also assess patients for the presence of other symptoms because they can contribute to or worsen nausea (thereby increasing distress in patients and their families).

Treatment

Before initiating pharmacologic therapy, clinicians should assess for and eliminate environmental stimuli. Treatment of the underlying cause, when identified, and stopping or reducing the dose on culprit drugs, where possible, also helps. With regard to drugs, selection of an agent based on the likely mechanism/active receptor type/ pathway (eg, ondansetron for 5 hydroxytryptamine-3 receptor mediated [5-HT$_3$]– mediated nausea, metoclopramide for D2-mediated nausea) is vital (**Table 3**). Also, consider using steroids to reduce tumor edema in the setting of either cortical nausea or visceral organ involvement and prokinetic agents for opioid-related and non– opioid-related delayed gastric emptying.

SUMMARY

The burden of nonpain symptoms such as anorexia, constipation, nausea, and vomiting contributes to patient suffering throughout the course of advanced illness. It is important to address symptom control throughout the disease trajectory, and especially at the end of life. Primary care clinicians must recognize these symptoms early, provide ongoing assessment, and keep abreast of evidence-based management strategies, including valid clinical protocols.

REFERENCES

1. Quill TE, Abernethy AP. Generalist plus specialist palliative care–creating a more sustainable model. N Engl J Med 2013;368:1173.
2. Schenker Y, Arnold R. Toward palliative care for all patients with advanced cancer. JAMA Oncol 2017;3:1459.
3. Available at: https://www.thectac.org/about/. Accessed October 7, 2018.
4. Bruera E. ABC of palliative care. Anorexia, cachexia, and nutrition. BMJ 1997; 315:1219.
5. Reville B, Axelrod D, Maury R. Palliative care for the cancer patient. Prim Care 2009;36(4):781–810.
6. Laviano A, Meguid MM, Rossi-Fanelli F. Cancer anorexia: clinical implications, pathogenesis, and therapeutic strategies. Lancet Oncol 2003;4:686–94.
7. Kalantar-Zadeh K, Block G, McAllister CJ, et al. Appetite and inflammation, nutrition, anemia, and clinical outcome in hemodialysis patients. Am J Clin Nutr 2004; 80:299.
8. Hughes CM, Woodside JV, McGartland C, et al. Nutritional intake and oxidative stress in chronic heart failure. Nutr Metab Cardiovasc Dis 2012;22:376.
9. Collins PF, Elia M, Stratton RJ. Nutritional support and functional capacity in chronic obstructive pulmonary disease: a systematic review and meta-analysis. Respirology 2013;18:616.

10. Cone RD. The central melanocortin system and energy homeostasis. Trends Endocrinol Metab 1999;10:211.

11. Elmquist JK. Anatomic basis of leptin action in the hypothalamus. Front Horm Res 2000;26:21.

12. Sleeman MW, Anderson KD, Lambert PD, et al. The ciliary neurotrophic factor and its receptor, CNTFR alpha. Pharm Acta Helv 2000;74:265.

13. Williams G, Harrold JA, Cutler DJ. The hypothalamus and the regulation of energy homeostasis: lifting the lid on a black box. Proc Nutr Soc 2000;59:385.

14. Woods SC, Schwartz MW, Baskin DG, et al. Food intake and the regulation of body weight. Annu Rev Psychol 2000;51:255.

15. Nakazato M, Murakami N, Date Y, et al. A role for ghrelin in the central regulation of feeding. Nature 2001;409:194.

16. Tschöp M, Smiley DL, Heiman ML. Ghrelin induces adiposity in rodents. Nature 2000;407:908.

17. Ahima RS, Flier JS. Leptin. Annu Rev Physiol 2000;62:413.

18. Friedman JM, Halaas JL. Leptin and the regulation of body weight in mammals. Nature 1998;395:763.

19. Wiffen PJ, Derry S, Moore RA. Impact of morphine, fentanyl, oxycodone or codeine on patient consciousness, appetite and thirst when used to treat cancer pain. Cochrane Database Syst Rev 2014;(5):CD011056.

20. Heckel M, Stiel S, Ostgathe C. Smell and taste in palliative care: a systematic analysis of literature. Eur Arch Otorhinolaryngol 2015;272:279.

21. Muscaritoli M, Anker SD. Consensus definition of sarcopenia, cachexia and pre-cachexia: joint document elaborated by Special Interest Group (SIG) "Cachexia-Anorexia in Chronic Wasting Diseases" and "Nutrition in Geriatrics". Clin Nutr 2010;29:154–9.

22. Morrison RS, Meier DE. Palliative care. N Engl J Med 2004;350(25):2582–90.

23. Higgins PD, Johanson JF. Epidemiology of constipation in North America: a systematic review. Am J Gastroenterol 2004;99:750.

24. Sandler RS, Drossman DA. Bowel habits in young adults not seeking health care. Dig Dis Sci 1987;32:841.

25. Potter J, Hami F, Bryan T, et al. Symptoms in 400 patients referred to palliative care services: prevalence and patterns. Palliat Med 2003;17:310–4.

26. Mancini I, Bruera E. Constipation in advanced cancer patients. Support Care Cancer 1998;6:356–64.

27. Johanson JF, Sonnenberg A, Koch TR. Clinical epidemiology of chronic constipation. J Clin Gastroenterol 1989;11:525–36.

28. Stewart WF, Liberman JN, Sandler RS, et al. Epidemiology of constipation (EPOC) study in the United States: relation of clinical subtypes to sociodemographic features. Am J Gastroenterol 1999;94:3530.

29. Solano JP, Gomes B, Higginson IJ. A comparison of symptom prevalence in far advanced cancer, AIDS, heart disease, chronic obstructive pulmonary disease and renal disease. J Pain Symptom Manage 2006;31:58.

30. Goodman M, Low J, Wilkinson S. Constipation management in palliative care: a survey of practices in the United Kingdom. J Pain Symptom Manage 2005;29:238–44.

31. American College of Gastroenterology Chronic Constipation Task Force. An evidence-based approach to the management of chronic constipation in North America. Am J Gastroenterol 2005;100(Suppl 1):S1.

32. Delgado Guay MO. Symptom Assessment. In: Yennurajalingam S, Bruera E, editors. Oxford American Handbook of Hospice and Palliative Medicine and Supportive Care. 2nd edition. New York: Oxford University Press; 2016. p. 13.
33. Reuben DB, Mor V. Nausea and vomiting in terminal cancer patients. Arch Intern Med 1986;146:2021.
34. Coyle N, Adelhardt J, Foley KM, et al. Character of terminal illness in the advanced cancer patient: pain and other symptoms during the last four weeks of life. J Pain Symptom Manage 1990;5:83.
35. Davis MP, Walsh D. Treatment of nausea and vomiting in advanced cancer. Support Care Cancer 2000;8:444.
36. Rhodes VA, McDaniel RW. Nausea, vomiting, and retching: complex problems in palliative care. CA Cancer J Clin 2001;51:232.
37. Gómez-Batiste X, Porta-Sales J, Espinosa-Rojas J, et al. Effectiveness of palliative care services in symptom control of patients with advanced terminal cancer: a spanish, multicenter, prospective, quasi-experimental, pre-post study. J Pain Symptom Manage 2010;40:652.
38. Tranmer JE, Heyland D, Dudgeon D, et al. Measuring the symptom experience of seriously ill cancer and noncancer hospitalized patients near the end of life with the memorial symptom assessment scale. J Pain Symptom Manage 2003;25:420.
39. Tsai JS, Wu CH, Chiu TY, et al. Symptom patterns of advanced cancer patients in a palliative care unit. Palliat Med 2006;20:617.
40. Blinderman CD, Homel P, Billings JA, et al. Symptom distress and quality of life in patients with advanced chronic obstructive pulmonary disease. J Pain Symptom Manage 2009;38:115.
41. Baines MJ. Nausea, vomiting and intestinal obstruction. BMJ 1997;315:1148–50.
42. National Comprehensive Cancer Network. Clinical practice guidelines in oncology. Antiemesis. Available at: http://www.nccn.org/professionals/physician_gls/PDF/antiemesis.pdf. Accessed October 29, 2018.
43. Kris MG, Hesketh PJ, Sommerfield MR, et al. American Society of Clinical Oncology guideline for antiemetics in oncology: update 2006. J Clin Oncol 2006;24(18):2932–47.
44. Wood GJ, Shega JW, Lynch B, et al. Management of intractable nausea and vomiting in patients at the end of life: "I was feeling nauseous all of the time … nothing was working". JAMA 2007;298:1196–207.
45. Dalal S, Del Fabbro E, Bruera E. Symptom control in palliative care. Part 1: oncology as a paradigmatic example. J Palliat Med 2006;9:391–408.

Communication Skills
Delivering Bad News, Conducting a Goals of Care Family Meeting, and Advance Care Planning

Caitlin N. Baran, MD[a],*, Justin J. Sanders, MD, MSc[b]

KEYWORDS

- Communication • Advance care planning • Goals of care
- Serious illness communication • Breaking bad news

KEY POINTS

- Clinicians face the difficult task of engaging patients in all stages of life and illness in communication about what goals and priorities should drive their medical decision making if they become very ill.
- Engaging patients in difficult communication is a necessary part of ensuring that patients obtain medical care that matches their goals and priorities.
- Prognosis should guide the content and timing of advance care planning tasks.
- Effective communication strategies and skills can help clinicians lead difficult conversations more effectively.
- Difficult communication tasks can be accounted for by using specific documentation and billing procedures.

Primary care clinicians face difficult conversations with patients across the life cycle. These conversations occur with patients young and old as they consider future adverse health states, receive bad news, and plan for future care in the setting of chronic or serious illness. Even the most skilled clinicians struggle to know what are the right words and the right times to engage patients in these conversations. This article focuses on practical communication skills to help clinicians lead difficult discussions more effectively. Because these conversations are enhanced by skills,

Disclosure Statement: J.J. Sanders is a faculty member in the Serious Illness Care Program at Ariadne Labs, which developed the Serious Illness Conversation Guide. C.N. Baran has nothing to disclose.
[a] Division of Geriatrics and Palliative Care, Massachusetts General Hospital, 55 Fruit Street, Boston, MA 02114, USA; [b] Department of Psychosocial Oncology and Palliative Care, Dana-Farber Cancer Institute, 450 Brookline Avenue, LW670, Boston, MA 02215, USA
* Corresponding author.
E-mail address: cbaran@mgh.harvard.edu

Prim Care Clin Office Pract 46 (2019) 353–372
https://doi.org/10.1016/j.pop.2019.05.003
0095-4543/19/© 2019 Elsevier Inc. All rights reserved.

strategies, and tools, it can be useful to think of them as procedures, for which adequate preparation is of paramount importance. These discussions are not singular events in a patient's care but parts of an evolving dialog across the health continuum (**Fig. 1**). As such, readers will discern overlap in skillful approaches to this communication throughout the life cycle.

OBJECTIVES

1. Describe the rationale for engaging patients in difficult conversations
2. Review strategies for engaging patients in difficult conversations across the life cycle
   a. Describe the use of prognosis as a framework for guiding clinicians in initiating these conversations
   b. Review communication techniques for navigating difficult conversations across the life cycle
3. Review essentials of workflow related to billing and documentation

WHY DIFFICULT COMMUNICATION IS CRITICAL

People get sick. When they do, the first person they may come to is their primary care clinician. These clinicians face the challenging task of shepherding a patient from presentation to diagnosis and treatment and through disease progression. Clinicians have the related task of helping patients plan for the eventuality of sickness, of eliciting from them information about whom they trust to make decisions when they cannot, and of clarifying their goals, values, and priorities. This planning has several benefits, including improved psychological well-being among patients and family members, and higher likelihood that patients will receive care that reflects what matters most to them.[1] By contrast, when clinicians fail to engage patients in difficult conversations that include prognostic disclosure, patients lose opportunities to plan and to focus on the things that matter most to them. They use treatments that are likely not to help.[2] They and their families suffer unnecessarily.[3,4]

PROGNOSIS AS A GUIDING FRAMEWORK FOR COMMUNICATION TIMING AND STRATEGIES

Prognosis, a word of Greek origin meaning "to know before," is used to describe a forecast of the likely course of a disease. The prognosis of a viral respiratory infection

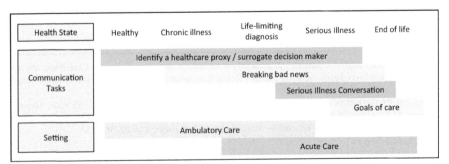

Fig. 1. Communication tasks by health state and setting. As patients face different states of health, clinicians will engage in corresponding communication tasks. These communication tasks occur in a variety of settings.

is resolution within 7 to 14 days. The prognosis of advanced metastatic pancreatic cancer is death within months to a year. Because it is a forecast with many variables, there is inherent uncertainty in prognostication. Despite this uncertainty, prognosis still has the potential to shape decision making because it creates a frame in which patients may consider and articulate their goals, values, and priorities. Not only does prognosis frame decision making for patients, it also provides a framework for clinicians to consider the timing and content of difficult communication tasks.[5]

PROGNOSTICATION CHALLENGES AND STRATEGIES
Formulating Prognosis

Communication about prognosis involves the communication of uncertainty. This uncertainty is reflective of the nature of human physiologic resilience and varied responses to therapy. Research demonstrates that clinicians exhibit systematic bias when estimating and communicating prognosis, some overestimating survival time by a factor of 5.[3,6] Undoubtedly this lack of precision contributes to provider discomfort in disclosing prognosis. However, despite both the discomfort and uncertainty, studies have shown both that patients want to hear prognosis and that they make different decisions about their care depending on the approximation of time.[7–9] The goal of prognostication is not to be right but rather to share expectations about what the future holds based on clinical information and within the context of varying degrees of uncertainty. Clinicians can use tools to enhance their understanding of a patient's risk of dying and disability. Clinical risk calculators, often available as online tools (listed in **Table 1**), use algorithms to determine the risk of death in a given time frame. When the relevant disease parameters are known, they can help clinicians formulate a prognosis. Another useful, though not highly sensitive, prognostic indicator is the so-called surprise question: "Would I be surprised if this patient died in the next year?" A "no" answer to the surprise question is highly predictive of mortality in patients with cancer and end-stage renal disease.[10] Beyond this screening question, using an assessment of the seriously ill patient's functional status, up-to-date data on disease progression, and subspecialist input about the trajectory of the patient's illness will help to develop a clearer picture of clinical prognosis.

Cultivating Prognostic Awareness

Experts have used the term "prognostic awareness" to describe a patient's understanding of their expected illness trajectory.[5] This awareness facilitates a patient's ability to engage in planning for the future. For example, a patient who expects many years left of life will likely set different goals, articulate different priorities, and make different treatment decisions than one who expects death within weeks to

Table 1	
Clinical prognostication tools	
Tool	**Application**
E-Prognosis (https://eprognosis.ucsf.edu/)[28]	Multiple medical conditions
Seattle Heart Failure Model[29]	Heart failure
BODE	Chronic obstructive pulmonary disease
MCI[a]	Dementia
Memorial Sloan Kettering Hospital Nonograms	Cancer

[a] Limited early data.

months. Prognostic awareness varies with time depending in part on the patient's ability to cope emotionally with prognostic information. Some patients want to avoid thinking or talking about prognosis whereas others are able to cognitively process the information but are too emotionally burdened to use it to make decisions: these patients have low prognostic awareness. Patients with high prognostic awareness are those who seem able to integrate and act on prognostic information. A normal pattern of coping for patients with serious illness has been described as a pendulum whereby patients vacillate between hopes that are more integrated with prognostic information, and thus more likely to be realized, and those that are less integrated and less likely to be realized (**Fig. 2**). This vacillation reflects a healthy and normal response to manage the emotional and cognitive load of difficult prognostic information.[11] A sense of urgency can arise for clinicians when patients with low prognostic awareness have higher short-term risk of death or disability. Later in this article, a stepwise approach is applied (**Fig. 3**) to cultivating prognostic awareness.

Difficult Communication Tasks Across the Life Cycle: A Case-Based Illustration

Here, a case-based approach is used to relate key communication tasks and strategies with different predictable health states across the life cycle. This case can be applied to patients with a variety of disease processes using prognosis to guide the timing and content of conversations. A list of communication skills and tools used in the illustrative case discussions is compiled in **Table 2**.

Healthy patient

James Monroe is a 20-year-old man who presents for a physical while on summer break from college. He has a medical history of mild intermittent asthma. James came out as gay to his parents this summer, straining his relationship with both of them, but particularly his father, Dave. He is closest with his older sister, Natasha.

Key Communication Task: Identify and assign a health care proxy.

Approach to the Communication Task: Clinicians may not readily consider that the identification of a surrogate decision maker is a priority for young, healthy patients. However, the biggest mortality risk factor for young adults is injury, which can leave them reliant on someone else to make decisions.[12] Therefore, although it may be

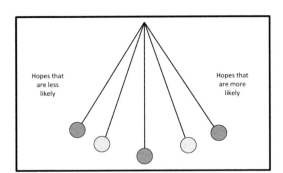

Fig. 2. Pendulum of prognostic awareness. The pendulum of awareness describes the phenomenon whereby as a part of healthy coping, patients vacillate between a more integrated understanding in which they articulate hopes that are more likely to be realized and a less integrated understanding in which they articulate hopes that are less likely to be realized. (*Adapted from* Jackson V, Jacobsen J, Greer J, et al. The cultivation of prognostic awareness through the provision of early palliative care in the ambulatory setting: a communication guide. J Palliat Med. 2013;16:894–900; with permission.)

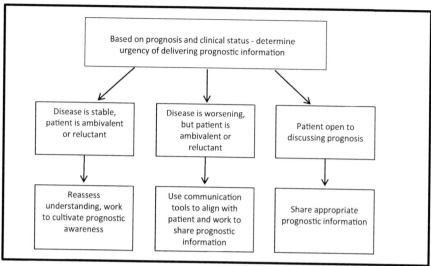

Fig. 3. Cultivating prognostic awareness. Once prognostic awareness has been assessed, clinicians can use this in conjunction with the prognosis to determine the pace with which prognostic awareness needs to be cultivated. (*Adapted from* Jackson V, Jacobsen J, Greer J, et al. The cultivation of prognostic awareness through the provision of early palliative care in the ambulatory setting: a communication guide. J Palliat Med. 2013;16:894–900; with permission.)

challenging for patients to engage in conversations about a catastrophic event for which they have little reference, it remains an important task. For all patients, the most important consideration when identifying a surrogate decision maker is the individual's trust in that person to make decisions that align with their goals, values, and priorities; thus, the nuances of relationships and family dynamics can and should affect selection of a surrogate. Patients should be encouraged to speak with their designated surrogate about health situations that they might find intolerable. One communication strategy that can aid this discussion is normalization, whereby the task is framed as normal for all individuals. **Box 1** illustrates a conversation in which a clinician engages James about assigning a health care proxy.

Patient with a new life-limiting diagnosis

Mr Dave Monroe, James's dad, is 53 years old when he presents to his primary care physician (PCP) to review a computed tomography (CT) scan showing evidence of metastatic colon cancer. Dave, who has a history of hypertension, presented 10 months ago with reports of intermittent rectal bleeding over the last 3 years. His PCP ordered a colonoscopy, which Dave deferred because of a busy work schedule. He presented to clinic last month with diffuse lower abdominal pain and 10-lb weight loss. He subsequently agreed to a CT scan and colonoscopy, the latter for next week.

Prognosis: Pending a further diagnostic workup, prognosis is uncertain. He is functionally well, which is important.

Key Communication Task: Breaking bad news.

Approach to the Communication Task: This is a turning point in the patient's health and in the clinician-patient relationship. These encounters can be intensely emotional for patients, which can hinder their ability to process and integrate information. Engaging with the emotional weight of serious news not only naturally builds rapport

Table 2
Additional tools for difficult communication

Challenge	Technique	Example
Responding to emotion	NURSE	See "Breaking bad news"
Responding to emotion	Simple and complex reflections	Simple reflection: Patient: *"I'm so sad"* Clinician: *"I hear you are really sad"* Complex reflection: Patient: *"I can't believe the medications didn't work"* Clinician: *"It must be really frustrating that this medicine wasn't helpful"*
Responding to emotion	Intentional silence	After delivering difficult news, such as *"I'm worried time is short,"* pausing intentionally allows space for the information to be processed and emotion to be realized
Ambivalence or reluctance	Talking about talking about it	Clinician: *""Do you have a sense of when it might be important to talk about this? How will you know it's the right time?"* …*"What are some advantages that you see to talking about the future? And what about disadvantages?"*… *"How might more information be helpful to you?"*
Ambivalence or reluctance	Box metaphor	Clinician: *"Talking about the future is like opening a box. There are times it's helpful to open the box and think and plan for the future. We don't always need to open the box, but we can decide together when it makes sense to do so"*
Ambivalence or reluctance	Consider a different state of health	Clinician: *"Have you had times where you have thought about what it might be like if you got sicker?"* Or *"I wonder if we should think together about what it would be like if you got sicker. It might be good to prepare in the event that did happen"*
Ambivalence or reluctance	Naming the dilemma	Clinician: *"I hear that you are hesitant to talk about the future, and on one hand I want to respect that, but on the other hand as your doctor I wouldn't be doing my job if I didn't talk to you about the possibility you might get sicker in the future"*
Ambivalence or reluctance	Use curiosity	Clinician: *"Can you tell me more about that?"*

(continued on next page)

Table 2
(continued)

Challenge	Technique	Example
Providing prognostic information	Permission statements	Clinician: *"Would it be okay if we talked about what we might expect with your illness in the future?"* When permission statements are met with a "no," use curiosity to explore this answer
Providing prognostic information	Hope-Worry-Wish Statements	Clinician: *"I hope the treatment helps you to feel better, but I worry that this may be the best you feel. I wish things were different."*

and demonstrates caring for the patient, it also sets the stage for cultivating prognostic awareness down the road. The "SPIKES" (Setting up, Perception, Invitation, Knowledge, Emotion, Summarize) model is one approach to navigating these conversations.[13]

SETTING UP:

Before the visit:

- Ask the patient to come in to discuss results of their workup, and ask that they bring support from family if possible
- Avoid giving information over the phone
- Ensure adequate visit time
- Gather information including the most likely diagnosis, general prognosis, treatment options, and next steps

At the visit:

- Arrange for privacy
- Involve significant others

Box 1
Health care proxy conversation

James, I hope you have a great year. There's one thing that I was hoping we could talk about.
  Sure Doc, What is it?

I wanted to talk with you about naming someone who could make decisions for you if something serious happened and you couldn't make medical decisions for yourself.
  Hey, I'm just going back to college. I play it pretty safe. I want to go medical school. Look, if something really bad happened, I don't want to be a vegetable.

I know you stay safe, and I can appreciate that you feel that way. That's a really unlikely scenario. But still, who would you trust to make medical decisions for you if you couldn't make them yourself?
  Well, I told you that things have been hard with my parents. I really trust my sister; I think she understands me. I can talk with her about anything, and I think she'll know what I want. Even though things have been hard, I also trust my mom. We don't really see eye to eye right now, but I think she'd make the right decisions. Is it good to have two people?

It is actually helpful to have an alternate person. This sounds like a good decision, James. Let's fill out a health care proxy form and we can revisit when you come back next year. You can always change your mind about who you think would be best to do this if necessary.

- Sit down
- Make connection with the patient
- Manage time constraints and interruptions

PERCEPTION: *Assess patient understanding.* In situations where other providers have been in contact with the patient it is helpful to elicit the patient's understanding of their illness stage.

INVITATION: *Ask permission to share information*: Although this may seem unnecessary, asking permission helps to empower patients and allows them to help guide the conversation.

KNOWLEDGE: Information sharing. This is the time to share the medical information you have gathered in a clear, concise manner. Using a "warning shot" to introduce difficult news may be helpful.[14]

EMOTION: *Respond to emotion.* Take time to acknowledge the emotional weight of this information. Responding to patient's emotions builds rapport, but also helps to create space and then cognitively process information.

The NURSE (Name, Understand, Respect, Support, Explore) acronym helps recall techniques for responding to emotion.[15] For example, if a patient says, *"I can't believe it's cancer…"*

Name the emotion: *"I can imagine this is shocking."*

Understand the emotion: *"It must be overwhelming to hear all of this news."*

Respect the patient: *"I'm amazed by the strength you've shown already as we've taken the steps to figure this out."*

Support the patient: *"I'll be here to help process all of this and we'll make a plan together."*

Explore the emotion: *"Can you tell me more about where your mind is?"*

Summarize: Take time at the end of the visit to summarize what you've discussed, to emphasize your alignment with the patient, and to delineate the next steps. Clinicians may recommend additional resources to support patients who are receiving bad news, such as social work, psychology, and chaplaincy. **Box 2** illustrates a "breaking bad news" conversation between a clinician and Mr Monroe.

Patient with a serious illness

Two years later, Dave is 55 years old. Following a difficult but ultimately helpful treatment for metastatic colon cancer, he has started to lose weight. A recent scan revealed cancer in the liver, lungs, and lymph nodes. Despite this, he is still working most days. He has had some abdominal pain and nausea, which are adequately managed with medications. Dave's oncologist has recommended a second-line cancer treatment. In a phone discussion the oncologist shares that he feels treatment is unlikely to provide the same response as the first one, and worries that the extent of recent progression signals an aggressive transformation of disease.

Prognosis: Dave's prognosis is likely months to a year, although it could be longer if he had another response to treatment. Given his disease process it is clinically appropriate to engage him in conversation about his serious illness and the care he may or may not want in the future.

Key Communication Task: Serious illness conversation.

Approach to Key Communication Task: These conversations between a clinician and a patient with a serious illness are a chance to elicit hopes and values and work together to plan for the future. Importantly, this is not an isolated conversation whereby a single plan is formulated, but rather a series of conversations to be revisited over time. **Fig. 4** contains a Serious Illness Conversation Guide (SICG), which provides focused language to be applied to this conversation.[16] Serious illness conversations

Box 2	
Breaking bad news	
Conversation	
Hi Dave, It's nice to see you. How have you been feeling?	
To be honest doctor, I've been kind of a wreck waiting for the results of that CT scan. So is my wife.	
I can imagine it's been really weighing on you. Is it okay if we talk about the results of the CT scan today?	Ask permission
Yes. Of course. That's the only thing on my mind.	
Did you want your wife to join you today?	
No, Carol's at work. Anyway, I wanted to come myself. Why, what's going on, doctor?	
It would be helpful if you told me what you're most worried about, Dave.	Assess perceptions
I'm really worried about cancer, doc. My brother died of cancer a few years ago.	
I remember you telling me that. Dave, I wish it was different, but the CT scan shows what looks like cancer that has spread to different places in your body.	Provide Information Wish statement
Oh god…I can't believe this.	
…	Intentional silence
I can imagine that this is really overwhelming to hear this news.	Acknowledge emotion
I don't know what to say.	
I'm here to help you process all this and to make a plan. Would it be helpful to take a minute to talk to Carol? Would it be helpful to do that together?	Affirm commitment
I appreciate that, doc. Man, I just can't believe it.	

present another chance to apply the general principles of "SPIKES" already discussed, while also applying the flow and language of the SICG as well as skills and techniques referenced in **Table 2**. The following reviews the broad approach to these conversations.

Part 1: setup, assessment of prognostic awareness, discussing prognosis The first part of a serious illness conversation entails establishing the frame in which goals, values, and priorities can be elicited from the patient and/or family. Doing so requires setting up the conversation in a way that feels psychologically safe for the patient (or surrogate), gaining a sense of their illness understanding and information preferences, and sharing a prognosis tailored to their information preferences. Assessing illness understanding creates a picture of how they are coping and their prognostic awareness. Respecting information preferences and asking permission fosters a sense of psychological safety for the patient. The Serious Illness Conversation Guide (see **Fig. 4**) provides examples of 3 different types of prognostic communication. Each step provides a foundation for the next.

Part 2: responding to emotion The second step involves using silence and other techniques to respond to the patient's emotions, which are inevitable and to be expected. Silence is a powerful form of nonverbal empathic communication. Being able to sit with and respond to emotion signals to patients the clinician's willingness to accompany them through difficult experiences. In addition, responding to emotion creates a space of psychological safety for the patient to process the weight of it, potentially helping to foster the positive coping skills that are associated with improved quality of life, and which may ultimately allow for cultivation of prognostic awareness.[17]

Serious Illness Conversation Guide

PATIENT-TESTED LANGUAGE

SET UP

"I'd like to talk about what is ahead with your illness and do some thinking in advance about what is important to you so that I can make sure we provide you with the care you want — **is this okay?**"

ASSESS

"What is **your understanding** now of where you are with your illness?"

"How much **information** about what is likely to be ahead with your illness would you like from me?"

SHARE

"I want to share with you **my understanding** of where things are with your illness..."

Uncertain: "It can be difficult to predict what will happen with your illness. I **hope** you will continue to live well for a long time but I'm **worried** that you could get sick quickly, and I think it is important to prepare for that possibility."
OR
Time: "I **wish** we were not in this situation, but I am **worried** that time may be as short as ___ (express as a range, e.g. days to weeks, weeks to months, months to a year)."
OR
Function: "I **hope** that this is not the case, but I **think** that this may be as good as you will feel, and things are likely to get more difficult."

EXPLORE

"What are your most important **goals** if your health situation worsens?"

"What are your biggest **fears and worries** about the future with your health?"

"What gives you **strength** as you think about the future with your illness?"

"What **abilities** are so critical to your life that you can't imagine living without them?"

"If you become sicker, **how much are you willing to go through** for the possibility of gaining more time?"

"How much does your **family** know about your priorities and wishes?"

CLOSE

"I've heard you say that ___ is really important to you. Keeping that in mind, and what we know about your illness, I **recommend** that we ___. This will help us make sure that your treatment plans reflect what's important to you."

"How does this plan seem to you?"

"I will do everything I can to help you through this."

Fig. 4. Serious illness conversation guide. (©2015 Ariadne Labs: A Joint Center for Health Systems Innovation (www.ariadnelabs.org) and Dana-Farber Cancer Institute. Revised April 2017. Licensed under the Creative Commons Attribution-NonCommercial-ShareAlike 4.0 International License, http://creativecommons.org/licenses/by-nc-sa/4.0.)

Part 3: exploring key topics and making a recommendation The third step involves eliciting goals, values, and priorities using a series of open-ended questions, followed by the formation of a recommendation for action that considers the patient's goals and the prognosis. Open-ended questions about what matters most to patients can provide a transition forward from the cognitive and emotional load of having shared prognostic information. The answers to these questions then frame the recommendation. Providing a recommendation can enhance psychological safety by providing a next step and closure to the conversation. It is necessary to recognize that the patient may have a variety of goals and hopes, but the recommendation should focus on the goals and hopes that are likely to be realized given the prognosis and treatment options, as illustrated in **Fig. 5.**

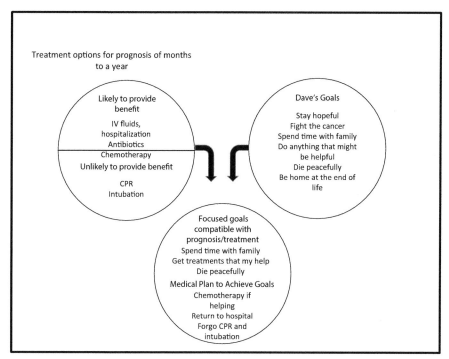

Fig. 5. Steps in providing a recommendation. Combining the patient's goals and values together with the treatment options for the given prognosis creates a framework for delivering a patient-centered recommendation. This recommendation reflects the values likely to be realized given the prognosis. The recommendation is discussed in terms of treatments that will be provided, and relevant interventions to forgo. (*Adapted from* Jacobsen J, Blinderman C, Alexander C, et al. "I'd recommend ..." how to incorporate your recommendation into shared decision making for patients with serious illness. J Pain Symptom Manage. 2018;55(4):1227; with permission.)

Boxes 3 and **4** illustrate the progression of a serious illness conversation over 2 visits with James Monroe. The first visit is a regular follow-up and the second occurs following a hospitalization.

Patient at the end of life

Five months later, Dave presents to the hospital with nausea, vomiting, and severe pain. He has a complete bowel obstruction. He has altered mental status and is confused and, at times, combative. This is his third hospitalization in 2 months. His chemotherapy has been on hold because of uncontrolled nausea, infections, and increasing debility. Dave has been spending most of his time in bed. The primary care clinician is asked to join the hospitalist for a family meeting with Carol, his wife, James, their son, and Natasha, their daughter. James has just started his first year in medical school. Nathasha is a stay-at-home mom with a newborn and a 2-year-old.

Prognosis: Dave's metastatic disease with declining functional status, multiple recent hospitalizations, and a new bowel obstruction complicated by altered mental status suggest a prognosis of days to weeks. His labs show hyponatremia and rising liver function test levels, with imaging showing extensive intrahepatic progression of disease.

Box 3	
Serious illness conversation, part 1	
Conversation	**Analysis**
Dave I'm hoping we could use some of our visit today to check in on how things are going and do some thinking in advance about what is important to you to make sure we provide you with the care you want. Would that be alright?	Set an agenda Ask permission
You know doc, I just try to stay positive and take it a day at a time. I don't think it helps to worry about the future—I'm just not a worrier. I'm young. I'm gonna beat this thing.	Ambivalence Low prognostic awareness
I appreciate staying positive and taking it a step at a time is important to you. This is a lot to go through and I admire your strength in facing it. I do wonder if it might be helpful at some point to think together about the future so we can make sure we have a plan in place to take care of you?	Reflect understanding Align with respect Consider the future
Maybe at some point, but not right now.	Reluctance
Do you have any thoughts about what the right time to do this might look like?	
Maybe once we see how this chemo works, then maybe we could.	
It can be overwhelming to talk about these things. Sometimes it's helpful to think about it like a box—sometimes it makes sense to open the box and talk about the future and plans we should make, and then close it and focus on other things. Knowing there's a plan for the future can actually help some people to focus more on the day to day.	Box metaphor
Yeah, I get that. I met with someone a while ago to make sure my pension is all squared away—so Carol is always taken care of. I get making practical plans.	
That's great that you were able to do that. I agree, I think we should make a time to think about some practical plans for the future at another visit would this be okay?	Encourage what advance care planning patient is doing Use the patient's language Plan to revisit conversation
Sure, that's fine.	

Key Communication Task: Goals of care discussion in a family meeting.

Approach to Key Communication Task: The strategies and approach discussed in the "serious illness" conversation can be applied here as well; however, there is the added nuance of working with a surrogate decision maker. There is also now clinical urgency necessitating that clinicians provide prognostic information and make treatment decisions.

UNIQUE CONSIDERATIONS FOR COMMUNICATION WITH FAMILIES

Clinicians are frequently faced with the task of communicating with a variety of family members. One of the particularly well-defined and challenging contexts is the family meeting for goals of care when the patient is too ill to participate. Experts have suggested that these family meetings prove challenging for clinicians for a few particular reasons[18]:

- Families bring the complexity of their own relationships and interactions to the meeting
- Each participant has his or her own interests
- Individuals have different emotional needs

| Box 4 |
| Serious illness conversation, part 2 |

Conversation	Analysis
Dave I'm glad you're feeling better after getting home for the hospital. I'm hoping we can take some time to do some of the practical planning we talked about a few weeks ago. Is that okay?	Set an agenda Ask permission to proceed
I guess now's as good of a time as ever these days.	Ambivalence
What's your sense of where things are right now with the cancer?	Assess illness understanding
Well, it's not great. The chemo didn't really do the job. So the cancer is spreading. But, like I said before I just need to keep positive.	Fair prognostic awareness
I definitely appreciate how important positivity is for you. That's my understanding as well. I know you see Dr Oh, the oncologist, but I want to check in and see how much information about what to expect going forward you'd like from me?	Assess information preferences
Well I trust you, I'd want to know whatever it is you know I think.	
I'm grateful for that. While I hope the next chemo is helpful, I am also worried that time could be shorter than we have been hoping. I hope it's not the case but I worry it could be as short as months to a year.	Provide prognostic information Hope/worry statement
Hangs head...But I was supposed to start the chemo next week. This is just unbelievable.	
I think that is still the best thing to do. I can imagine this is overwhelming.	Acknowledge emotion
It's not what I was hoping to hear.	
I wish it were different. I'm going to continue to be here for you, I want you to know that. Dave, can I ask what would be important to you if you were to get sicker?	Wish statement Affirm nonabandonment Ask permission Identify what's important
You know me. I just want to spend my time working on my cars and being with Carol....Actually, I'd really like to patch things up with James. I guess if it was really bad I'd just want to be home, just with everyone.	
It's really helpful to hear how you'd think about things. Are there certain things that feel so critical to you that you couldn't live without them?	Identify critical abilities
I don't think I could handle it if I couldn't talk with my family.	
Knowing you, that makes sense to me. Dave, Would it be helpful to hear some recommendations about how we best take care of you going forward?	Ask permission
Absolutely doc	
I recommend that we continue with the plan for chemotherapy next week, and that we keep checking in about how it's going. I think it makes sense to continue to treat anything we can readily fix and work on everything we can to help you live well. I also want to recommend that we put a plan in place should you get acutely ill. I would recommend that given the cancer and what's important to you that we forgo interventions that are unlikely to help, which at this time would include cardiopulmonary resuscitation—instead we would allow for a peaceful passing when that time comes.	Offer recommendation
Gosh, I hadn't thought about most of that. It sounds like we keep doing things but when it's my time it's my time? That sounds right to me doc.	

- Preferences for decision making may differ
- There may be disagreement about the best course of action

Using a variety of communication skills particular to family meetings can help to ease these challenges for the clinician. These techniques are identified in **Table 3**.

In addition to using communication techniques it is also helpful to acknowledge the complexity of family dynamics.[19] Returning to the case, while James's wife and each of his kids individually bring a different experience and perspective, when they are together as a family the result is more than just the sum of their experiences and perspectives. The role each individual plays within the family, and the relationships among each other, shape the way the family will make decisions.[19] Dave's role as a "provider" for his family, his strained relationship with his son James, and James's close relationship with Natasha are just a few of the dynamics that will play a part in a family meeting with the Monroe family. **Box 5** illustrates a goals of care family meeting with the Monroes.

Cross-Cultural Communication

Patients from marginalized and underserved communities often experience difficult conversations within a context of mistrust. This mistrust results from both negative personal and family experiences with health care systems and providers, as well as historical inequities in access to high-quality care and unethical experimentation at the hands of medical providers and the government. These issues can be particularly salient when discussing treatment options near the end of life, especially when individuals feel the covert pressure of societal norms that favor limitations to life-sustaining treatments. Without covering the myriad of issues that can arise when

Table 3
Additional strategies to apply in family meetings

Challenge	Technique	Example
Burden of decision making	Apply principle of substituted judgment	Clinician: "If he could talk with us now how would he answer this question?"
Hierarchy of family decision making	Consider family dynamics	Clinician: "How do you all make decisions like this as a family?"
Difference of opinion among family	Naming the disagreement	Clinician: "It sounds like you each have different ideas about what he would prefer"
Disruptive family member	Remain neutral	Clinician: "It's important to me to hear from each of you"
Emotionally charged	Acknowledge the emotion	Clinician: "This must be so sad for you as a family"
General tool for approaching family meetings	Value	Value: "I appreciate you coming today. Hearing from you all helps us to better care for __" Acknowledge: "This is difficult news" Listen and understand: "Tell me about what life was like for __ more recently. What was important to him? What would he say if we could talk to him now?"

Box 5	
Family meeting for goals of care	
Conversation	**Analysis**
Thank you all for being here. I'd like to spend some time talking about where things stand with Dave's illness and thinking together about what makes sense in caring for him going forward. Would that be okay with you all?	Value family Set an agenda Ask permission to proceed
Carol: We're happy to be here. We would do anything for Dave.	
Are there other things you all would like to make sure we also talk about today?	Understand family agenda
James: We want to hear the results from his labs today too.	
We will be sure to talk about the latest results. To help me know what other information will be helpful, I'd like to start by asking, what's your understanding of where things are with Dave's illness?	Assess prognostic awareness
Carol: Well we know he has the cancer and that it's been spreading more. He's been having a harder time at home recently. We know he's sick really sick, but we're hoping he'll shake this. "Stay positive" that's what Dave says.	Good prognostic awareness
Natasha: He did okay for a while with the chemo, but he's felt so bad the last couple times he couldn't get it at those appointments.	Fair prognostic awareness
James: His cancer is progressing because he can't get the chemotherapy, but maybe there's another chemo with less side effects that he could get to give him more time.	Low prognostic awareness
I can imagine these last months have been really hard as he's been in the hospital more. It sounds like you all understand that he has gotten sicker. I also hear that maintaining hope has been important. I'd like to share some more medical information about where things stand now if that would be okay.	Acknowledge difficulty Complex reflection Ask permission
James: yes, let's hear the labs and any other results you've gotten	
Dave came in with vomiting and confusion. Since then we have found he has a bowel obstruction. We also saw the cancer has increased in his liver. His labs show worsening liver function. All of this together has made him quite confused. Given this and how much strength he's lost recently I am worried time could be as short as days to weeks.	Share prognosis Hope/worry statement Pause after sharing prognosis
Carol: Tearful	
James: Well we can't just give up. He's young. I want him to get everything you've got!	Consider family dynamics/ relationships
I know that this is not the news any of you were hoping for today. I can appreciate that Dave would want to receive any therapy that might be helpful to him. Dave is so sick right now that more chemotherapy would be likely to cause him more harm than good.	Appreciate patient values
James: We just need to stay positive like dad always says.	Reluctance
Carol: I think that's right, maybe he just needs more time.	Reluctance
On one hand I know this is really difficult to talk about and that staying positive is important. On the other hand I am worried things are changing quickly medically and we need to be prepared. Would it be okay if we talked more about what it would be like if things don't go as we hope?	Name the dilemma
Natasha: I think we need to be prepared. We don't want him to suffer.	

James: I guess so.

I know staying positive is important to Dave. Can you all tell me given that time is likely shorter than we'd hope, if Dave could talk to us right now what would he say is most important?	Identify what's most important
Carol: We've talked about this before, he'd just want to be with the kids.	
Natasha: He wouldn't want to suffer. He's been through so much. He'd never want to be like he is in that room right now—he doesn't know what's going on half the time.	
James: Yeah, he'd want to be home. But if there was anything else that could be done he'd want that too.	
It sounds like being comfortable is important to him and being home if possible. I also hear that if we thought there was a treatment that would be helpful he would want to pursue that. This is such a hard situation. I wonder if it might be helpful to hear a recommendation about how we might best take care of Dave going forward.	Summarize Offer recommendation
Carol: That would be so helpful. He's always trusted you.	
Given that time may be short and Dave would prioritize being with family and being peaceful at the end of life I would recommend that we focus our treatments on things that will keep him comfortable. I would recommend we put a plan in place to get him home if possible while focusing on managing symptoms and avoiding coming back to the hospital. I think it would be helpful to have all the resources available to support this plan, which would also include hospice. What are your thoughts about this plan?	Make recommendation
Carol: Tearful. I was worried this was coming. But Dave and I have known, and I know that's what he's wanted.	
James: Mom. You can't just give up like that. He'd want to fight.	
James it sounds like you might have a different idea of what your dad might want, is that right?	Name the disagreement
James: I don't know. (Tearful) I just don't want him to go.	
It's heartbreaking to be thinking about these things. I know how much you care about your dad.	Acknowledge emotion Value family
James: I do. We all do. How do we get him home with hospice then?	
We will work together with other team members to get the process moving. We will keep taking care of Dave and supporting you all as family.	Affirm commitment

advance care planning or discussing goals of care, it is noteworthy that socioculturally sensitive communication effectively uses open-ended questions about patients' goals, values, and priorities as an effective starting place for initiating conversations of this type, as they demonstrate respect and build rapport. By contrast, conversations that take as a starting place the treatments themselves are likely to engender or perpetuate mistrust.

Billing and Documentation

Documentation should include a list of those present for the conversation as well as a general summary of the encounter, including, where possible, direct quotes that help illuminate the patient's goals, values, and priorities that may inform any future treatment decisions. To make such information useful at multiple points of care, clinicians should, when possible, use structured advance care planning models in the electronic health record to document patient preferences. **Box 6** is an example of this for Dave.

Formal documents

Health care proxy form or durable power of attorney of health care: As already noted, this form identifies the patient's health care decision maker. Individual states regulate the process for identifying a surrogate decision maker for those without an official documented health care proxy.

Orders for life-sustaining treatment (POLST/MOLST/COLST/MOST): These medical orders (POLST, physician orders for life-sustaining treatment; MOLST, medical orders for life-sustaining treatment; COLST, clinician orders for life-sustaining treatment; MOST, medical orders for scope of treatment) document specific preferences regarding a range of life-sustaining treatments, ranging from resuscitation and intubation, to hospitalization, receipt of antibiotics, and hemodialysis. *These are the only legally binding documents for DNR (do not resuscitate) outside of the hospital*. These forms were designed for use by patients who are thought to be within the last year of life. Evidence suggests that POLST forms may enhance the delivery of goal-concordant care.[20–23]

Advanced directives: Living wills (also called health care or medical directives) are legal documents that vary widely in content and may differ by state; some focus on "general wishes about medical care" whereas others provide detailed specifications for or against specific interventions. They are not a legal order to prevent or ensure resuscitation, and evidence fails to support their effective use in delivering care outlined therein.[23–25]

Billing

The first step in billing for these conversation procedures is to discern whether the conversation comprised "advance care planning" or "counseling and care coordination." In this article, assigning a health care proxy, having a conversation about serious illness, and leading a family meeting for goals of care would all fall under "advance care planning."[26] **Box 7** contains steps for this billing procedure. The office visit to discuss a new life-limiting diagnosis represents a visit in which it is likely that >50% of time is spent on counseling and coordination of care, suggesting the use of a

---

Box 6
Example of documentation of goals of care conversation

Document summation of conversations:

Illness understanding: Dave understands his cancer is not curable and treatment is palliative.

Hopes/values: Hoping for more time with his family. He values his independence and his ability to remain mentally clear so he can interact with his kids and grandkids. He hopes for a peaceful passing when it's his time.

Worries: Concerned about losing his independence and his family needing to care for him.

Preferences for care at this time: Continue chemotherapy in hopes of controlling cancer. Continue to treat all potentially reversible illness. Prioritize being home at end of life if possible.

Recommendations discussed: Recommended continuing chemotherapy and treating those things we can reverse. Recommended social work support for him and his family. Recommended forgoing cardiopulmonary resuscitation in the event he gets much sicker given values discussed today. Dave is accepting of all of these recommendations.

Box 7
Billing for advance care planning

What: *Face-to-face* discussions with patients/health care provider about goals, values, and preferences to direct medical decision making. Includes the explanation and discussion of advance directives (+/− completion of a form)

Basics:
- Document total time
- Can bill on same day as E&M
  ○ Advance care planning time MUST be separate
  ○ Use 25 modifier
- As frequent as medically indicated
  ○ Initial conversation
  ○ Change in serious illness
  ○ Change in goals
- Service provided by MD, NP, or PA

Documentation:
- Account of discussion, including nature of advance care planning
  ○ Discussion of prognosis
  ○ Discussion of goals in relation to medical decision making
  ○ Code status
  ○ Health care proxy
- Who was present (providers and patient/family members)
- Total time spent in face-to-face encounter (time in/time out NOT needed)
- 99497: First 16 minutes of advance care planning discussion
- 99498: each additional 30 minutes (start using at minute 31)

---

time-based level of service.[27] Recognizing that patients also have acute issues that may be addressed during the visit, such as symptoms, it may still be appropriate to bill based on complexity if the necessary requirements are met on HPI, ROS, and examination. Of note, an E&M (Evaluation & Management) code can be billed on the same visit as that of an advanced care plan if performed and documented as separately identifiable services.

CLOSING THOUGHTS

Advances in medicine and the ever-changing landscape of health care delivery demand that health systems and clinicians increase their capacity to engage patients in high-quality communication. Although patients receive care from a variety of clinicians in a multitude of subspecialties, primary care clinicians are often uniquely positioned to provide care continuity through health and illness. This article highlights practical communication skills and strategies to be applied when caring for patients across the life cycle. Clinicians should apply and adapt these tools to fit their own style and the needs of patients. Along with the challenges inherent to engaging patients in these difficult conversations comes the profound reward of doing the right thing for patients to ensure that they receive the best care possible.

REFERENCES

1. Temel JS, Greer JA, Muzikansky A, et al. Early palliative care for patients with metastatic non-small-cell lung cancer. N Engl J Med 2010;363(8):733–42.
2. Weeks JC. Relationship between cancer patients' predictions of prognosis and their treatment preferences. JAMA 1998;279(21):1709.

3. A controlled trial to improve care for seriously ill hospitalized patients. The study to understand prognoses and preferences for outcomes and risks of treatments (SUPPORT). The SUPPORT Principal Investigators. JAMA 1995;274(20):1591–8.

4. Steinhauser KE, Christakis NA, Clipp EC, et al. Factors considered important at the end of life by patients, family, physicians, and other care providers. JAMA 2000;284(19):2476–82.

5. Jackson VA, Jacobsen J, Greer JA, et al. The cultivation of prognostic awareness through the provision of early palliative care in the ambulatory setting: a communication guide. J Palliat Med 2013;16(8):894–900.

6. Parkes CM. Accuracy of predictions of survival in later stages of cancer. Br Med J 1972;2(5804):29–31.

7. Yun YH, Lee CG, Kim S, et al. The attitudes of cancer patients and their families toward the disclosure of terminal illness. J Clin Oncol 2004;22(2):307–14.

8. Kaplowitz SA, Campo S, Chiu WT. Cancer patients' desires for communication of prognosis information. Health Commun 2002;14(2):221–41.

9. Dupree CY. The attitudes of black Americans toward advance directives. J Transcult Nurs 2000;11(1):12–8. Available at: http://graphics.tx.ovid.com/ovftpdfs/FPDDNCGCGAPDCL00/fs046/ovft/live/gv023/00002045/00002045-2000 01000-00004.pdf.

10. Gómez-Batiste X, Martínez-Muñoz M, Blay C, et al. Utility of the NECPAL CCOMS-ICO© tool and the Surprise Question as screening tools for early palliative care and to predict mortality in patients with advanced chronic conditions: a cohort study. Palliat Med 2017;31(8):754–63.

11. Weisman AD. On dying and denying: a psychiatric study of terminality. New York: Behavioral Publications; 1972.

12. National vital statistics reports: Center for Disease Control and Prevention. 2018. Available at: https://www.cdc.gov/nchs/products/nvsr.htm. Accessed October 18, 2018.

13. Baile WF, Buckman R, Lenzi R, et al. SPIKES—a six-step protocol for delivering bad news: application to the patient with cancer. Oncologist 2000;5(4):302–11.

14. Patvardhan C. Breaking bad news. BMJ 2005;330(7500):1131.

15. Portenoy RK, Bruera E, editors. Topics in palliative care. New York: Oxford University Press; 1997.

16. Bernacki RE, Block SD. American College of Physicians High Value Care Task Force. Communication about serious illness care goals: a review and synthesis of best practices. JAMA Intern Med 2014;174(12):1994–2003.

17. Greer JA, Jacobs JM, El-Jawahri A, et al. Role of patient coping strategies in understanding the effects of early palliative care on quality of life and mood. J Clin Oncol 2018;36(1):53–60.

18. Back A, Arnold RM, Tulsky JA, editors. Mastering communication with seriously ill patients: balancing honesty with empathy and hope. Cambridge (England): Cambridge University Press; 2009.

19. King DA, Quill T. Working with families in palliative care: one size does not fit all. J Palliat Med 2006;9(3):704–15.

20. Bomba PA, Kemp M, Black JS. POLST: An improvement over traditional advance directives. Cleve Clin J Med 2012;79(7):457–64.

21. Pedraza SL, Culp S, Falkenstine EC, et al. POST forms more than advance directives associated with out-of-hospital death: insights from a state registry. J Pain Symptom Manage 2016;51(2):240–6.

22. Tolle SW, Tilden VP, Nelson CA, et al. A prospective study of the efficacy of the physician order form for life-sustaining treatment. J Am Geriatr Soc 1998;46(9): 1097–102.

23. Teno JM, Licks S, Lynn J, et al. Do advance directives provide instructions that direct care? SUPPORT Investigators. Study to Understand Prognoses and Preferences for Outcomes and Risks of Treatment. J Am Geriatr Soc 1997;45(4): 508–12. Available at: http://www.ncbi.nlm.nih.gov/pubmed/9100722.

24. Fisch MJ. Advance directives: sometimes necessary but rarely sufficient. JAMA Oncol 2015. https://doi.org/10.1001/jamaoncol.2015.2074.

25. Teno JM. Advance directives: time to move on. Ann Intern Med 2004;141(2): 159–60. Available at: http://www.ncbi.nlm.nih.gov/pubmed/15262674.

26. Frequently asked questions about billing the Physician Fee Schedule for advance care planning services. 2016. Available at: https://www.cms.gov/Medicare/Medicare-Fee-for-Service-Payment/PhysicianFeeSched/Downloads/FAQ-Advance-Care-Planning.pdf. Accessed October 22, 2018.

27. Evaluation and Management Services. 2017. Available at: https://www.cms.gov/Outreach-and-Education/Medicare-Learning-Network-MLN/MLNProducts/Downloads/eval-mgmt-serv-guide-ICN006764.pdf.

28. E-Prognosis calculators. Available at: https://eprognosis.ucsf.edu/. Accessed October 21, 2018.

29. Seattle Heart Failure Model. Available at: https://depts.washington.edu/shfm. Accessed October 21, 2018.

Psychosocial Issues and Bereavement

E. Alessandra Strada, PhD, MSCP

KEYWORDS

- Bereavement • Grief • Palliative care • Psychosocial care • Emotional distress
- Caregiver burden • End of life

KEY POINTS

- Patients with serious illness and their family caregivers face many ongoing psychosocial challenges caused by the impact of the disease process on function, mood, coping, relationships, and overall quality of life.
- Because poorly managed pain and symptoms can cause severe distress that mimics psychiatric disorders, it is essential that optimal symptom management be achieved before diagnosing depression or anxiety.
- Establishing a trusting relationship with the patient and the family requires clinicians to provide culturally competent care that conveys respect for cultural preferences regarding communication style, expression of grief, approach to medical decisions, and ways of coping with distress.
- The grieving process is a normal and expected part of the illness experience for patients and family caregivers and should not be pathologized, but should be supported and monitored for development of complications (ie, prolonged grief disorder, major depression, and anxiety disorders).

INTRODUCTION

Patients with serious illness and their family caregivers face numerous ongoing psychological and social concerns and stressors throughout the disease trajectory. These stressors can negatively affect mood, cognitive function, interpersonal relationships, and medical decision making. If not recognized and adequately addressed, these challenges can seriously undermine coping and resilience, eroding psychological well-being and quality of life.

Because each patient and family system are unique, their response and adaptation to the challenges of living with serious illness are influenced by multiple factors rooted in personal history and psychosocial and cultural context. These factors determine how they make meaning of the illness, how they make medical decisions honoring

Disclosure: The author has nothing to disclose.
Psychopharmacology Program, Alliant University, San Francisco, CA, USA
E-mail address: astrada23@gmail.com

Prim Care Clin Office Pract 46 (2019) 373–386
https://doi.org/10.1016/j.pop.2019.05.004
0095-4543/19/© 2019 Elsevier Inc. All rights reserved.

core values, how they understand and cope with distress, how they preserve valued relationships and connections along the disease trajectory, and how they preserve their sense of personal dignity. A psychosocial assessment allows providers to understand fully is the patient and the family living with the disease. In patient and family–centered care, "It's much more important to know what sort of patient has a disease than what sort of disease a patient has."[1] This point is especially poignant and relevant in palliative care, which addresses patient and family concerns and needs at the most vulnerable and distressing time. The psychosocial assessment should be understood as an ongoing process and conducted at every encounter to monitor coping of existing challenges and detect the presence of new stressors.

APPROACHING PSYCHOSOCIAL ISSUES WITH CULTURAL COMPETENCE

A trusting relationship with medical providers is a fundamental first step that allows the patient and family caregivers to share what matters most to them, what they are struggling with, what they fear, and how they are coping. Further, a trusting relationship requires the provider to be familiar with the patient's and family's cultural values and to communicate validation and respect. Beyond ethnicity and group affiliation, culture includes beliefs systems, practices, and core values that they share with a particular group and others that are unique to them.

To address any psychosocial issues effectively, whether anxiety or depression, communication challenges, or family conflict, it is necessary to understand the patient and family core cultural values and the ways in which they affect experience, behavior, and decision making.[2] Rather than assuming the patient's and the family's cultural values, the provider must explore them by asking open-ended questions and allowing the patient and family to educate the physician about what is important to them.

It should be noted that every patient-provider encounter is a cross-cultural encounter, because it involves communication and negotiation between at least 4 cultural entities:

- Culture of medicine
- Culture of the medical system
- Culture of the patient and the family
- Culture of the physician

The culture of medicine and the culture of the medical system are represented by different sets of values and practices that may be in conflict with each other. In a more general meaning, the culture of medicine involves approaches and values related to diagnosing and managing disease respecting patient autonomy and self-determination. In contrast, the culture of the medical system is defined by values and practices that are focused on delivery of care and financial sustainability.

The 2 cultures can result in different sets of priorities that may clash in the daily reality of the clinical encounter. For example, the need to see a certain number of patients a day and comply with documentation during the encounter is part of the culture of the medical system. In contrast, the culture of medicine in its more holistic expression focuses on good communication with the patient and the family, especially in the context of serious illness. Furthermore, each primary care provider may also have a personal culture that places great value on establishing a personal connection with individual patients by listening carefully to their stories and using the clinical encounter as an opportunity for providing support, and may feel frustrated by having little time available for exploration of psychosocial concerns. Similarly, the patients and families may avoid sharing challenges they are facing, because a short clinical encounter may not allow for enough safety and psychological comfort.

Although it is not expected that medical providers function as therapists, those who are able to find a way to explore the psychosocial domain during each encounter can add greatly to the patients' and families' well-being. They can offer continuity and comfort even in the midst of chaos and distress.

COMMON PSYCHOSOCIAL STRESSORS FOR PATIENTS AND FAMILY CAREGIVERS

Common psychosocial concerns for the patients and the families are related to several areas: the challenges of managing the disease by navigating the medical system, managing psychological stresses and psychiatric complications, coping with existential and spiritual concerns, managing practical and social stressors, and preserving family relationships in the context of role changes and caregiving (**Table 1**).

Managing the Disease and Navigating the Medical System

Living with serious illness is characterized by unwelcome change and the necessity to make important and complex decisions about medical care and continue functioning. This creates ongoing stress for the patients and family caregivers, requiring them to constantly adapt to new circumstances caused by the evolution of the disease process.[3] In order to maintain a sense of well-being, they can adapt to the changes by redefining a new normal after every physical, psychological, or social change. Abrupt and unexpected changes (eg, the need to stop active treatment because of severe adverse effects; presence of acute complications that significantly change prognosis) take a major toll on psychological defenses. Every change that affects the patient's function can negatively affect the ability to cope and can create anxiety and hopelessness.

Coping with Social Stressors

The negative impact of financial and practical stressors cannot be overstated, because it can compromise coping even in resilient patients and families. If not asked

Table 1 Common psychosocial stressors for patients and family caregivers	
Disease Management	• Participate in medical decision making • Navigate the medical system • Deal with constant change and need for adaptation finding a new normal
Social	• Deal with possible financial challenges caused by loss of job, health insurance issues, transportation, housing problems • Deal with discrimination, racism, inequality, poverty • Concerns about impact of immigration status • Communicate with medical providers to ensure cultural practices, preferences, and values are understood, respected, and supported
Family/Interpersonal	• Preserve family function during caregiving • Manage caregiver burden
Psychological/Psychiatric	• Cope with ongoing grieving process during illness • Manage new psychiatric complications; eg, depression, anxiety • Manage exacerbation form prior psychiatric disorders; eg, personality disorders, psychotic disorder, substance use disorder • Cope with grief during bereavement

directly about any financial or practical challenges, many individuals who were self-reliant do not disclose distress, because of a sense of shame and personal pride.

Vulnerable populations, including sexual and ethnic minorities, face significant challenges accessing adequate health care services and receiving adequate psychosocial support.[4,5] They are often victims of discrimination and bias. Fear of deportation or being separated from family because of immigration or legal status can create major distress and negatively affect the ability to participate in medical treatment. Lesbian, gay, or bisexual patients with cancer have reported experiencing isolation and significant financial and health insurance coverage challenges during and after medical treatment.[6,7]

Preserving Family Relationships During Caregiving

The continual energy expenditure required to manage and live with serious illness can destabilize the entire family system by forcing role changes and introducing new and demanding physical tasks of caregiving.[8] Family caregivers may not be forthcoming in describing their own challenges and presence of caregiver burden. They may be afraid of being considered inadequate caregivers or may be concerned that, by attracting attention to themselves, they may detract from the focus on the patient. However, undetected caregiver distress results in increased caregiver burden and sense of being overwhelmed. This situation can compromise the physical and psychological safety and well-being of both patient and family caregiver. Therefore, assessment and intervention in this area must be thorough and ongoing.[9]

Managing Psychological Challenges and Psychiatric Complications

It has become well recognized that poorly managed pain can create severe distress that can mimic or even cause depression and anxiety. The effective management of psychosocial issues always requires adequate management of pain and other physical symptoms. Any new psychiatric diagnosis (eg, depression) should be deferred in the context of undermanaged pain and revisited after adequate medical management has been achieved.

Assessment and management of depression

Depressive symptoms are a common expression of distress in patients with serious illness and can range from occasional low mood to a diagnosis of major depression. Patients and family caregivers commonly report moments of profound sadness and difficulty coping with the stresses of serious illness. These reactions are especially common after receiving additional bad news after initial diagnosis (eg, disease recurrence or worsening, ineffectiveness of treatment).

Mood variations are a normal response and typical of a normal grieving process. When sadness and depressive symptoms are part of normal grieving, mood fluctuates and the patient or family caregiver can still experience moments of positive connection with loved ones and a sense of personal meaning. The key here is fluctuation.

However, mood that does not fluctuate and is depressed every day, most of the day, causing significant impairment and suffering, indicates the presence of major depression. Patients and family caregivers with undertreated major depression experience reduced quality of life, increased suicidal ideation, and desire for hastened death.

Recognizing the difference between a normal grieving process (during illness and in bereavement) and major depression can be challenging, because even normal grieving causes intense distress (**Box 1**).

> **Box 1**
> **Difference between grieving and major depression**
>
> Grieving
>
> - Mood fluctuates alternating moments of distress and isolation with ability to connect with loved ones
> - Severe symptoms, for example suicidal thoughts are fleeting or transient
> - Distress is caused by the thought of leaving loved ones (in patients) or by the death of the loved one (in bereaved caregivers)
> - The griever feels comforted by receiving social support
>
> Major depression
>
> - Persistent depressed mood may include suicidal ideation
> - Mood does not fluctuate even after positive events; for example, visits from loved ones
> - Negative and ruminative thought process
> - Feelings of worthlessness and self-deprecation
> - Mood does not improve with social support

Although it is not a normal consequence of illness, major depression is prevalent in serious illness and remains under-recognized and undertreated because of professional and attitudinal barriers:

- Belief that depression is a normal response in advanced illness
- Fear of pathologizing end of life
- Concerns about adding to the symptom burden by prescribing psychotropic medication
- Diagnostic difficulties caused by overlap of neurovegetative symptoms in depression and advanced illness

The reported prevalence of major depression in advanced cancer ranges from 3% to 58% based on the different thresholds of assessment tools. Major depression is highly prevalent in pancreatic cancer, advanced heart failure, chronic obstructive pulmonary disease, end-stage renal disease, and end-stage acquired immunodeficiency syndrome.[10,11]

Risk factors for depression include a prior history of depression, inadequate pain and symptom management, and metabolic and endocrinologic abnormalities. Depression is also associated with the use of corticosteroids, β-blockers, and certain chemotherapy agents.

Persistent low mood and decreased interest in previously valued activities are considered hallmarks of depression. Somatic symptoms of depression include fatigue, decreased ability to concentrate, psychomotor retardation, hypersomnia, and weight loss. Because these symptoms are also common manifestations of advanced illness, accurate diagnosis of depression in the seriously ill can be challenging. Therefore, the diagnostic focus should be on psychological symptoms:

- Depressed appearance
- Social withdrawal and decreased talkativeness
- Ruminative negative self-talk
- Guilt, sense of worthlessness, self-pity
- Pessimism

- Hopelessness
- Lack of reactivity.

Depression increases the risk for suicidal ideation, with known risk factors being:

- Depression and hopelessness
- Unmanaged pain and physical symptoms
- Cognitive dysfunction and delirium
- Poor social support
- Prior history of psychiatric illness
- Prior suicide attempts
- Spiritual and existential distress

The presence of suicidal risk should always be assessed by determining the presence of:

- Suicidal ideation
- Suicidal plan
- Intent
- Availability of means to complete the suicidal plan

It is important to ask the patient or the family caregiver clearly and directly whether they have been thinking about ending their lives. This question allows the provider to determine risk level and appropriate interventions.[12] There is no evidence to support the concern that patients or family caregivers will become more distressed or will begin thinking about suicide if asked openly.

Pharmacologic and Psychological Management

Depression is not a normal development in serious illness, even at end of life. Because it causes a decreased quality of life in patients and family caregivers, it should always be treated. Based on the patient's level of function, prognosis, and personal preferences, treatment can be pharmacologic, psychological/behavioral, or both.

Pharmacologic management of depression in patients with advanced illness has not been thoroughly studied. However, several randomized trials and meta-analyses indicate the effectiveness of antidepressants. Antidepressants are chosen based on side effect profile, available time for treatment, target symptom, and coexisting medical problems. Selective serotonin reuptake inhibitors (SSRIs; citalopram, escitalopram, sertraline) are generally considered first-line treatment because of a more favorable side effect profile. Serotonin norepinephrine reuptake inhibitors (SNRIs; duloxetine, venlafaxine) are often selected for depressed patients who are also experiencing neuropathic pain. Tricyclics may be more effective for severely depressed patients but have a less favorable side effect profile. The use of stimulants can promote improvement in mood and energy within 24 to 48 hours and may be appropriate to relieve some depressive symptoms in patients with a prognosis of weeks. The chosen pharmacologic agent should be started at the lowest possible dose and increased slowly while carefully monitoring tolerability of adverse effects.[13]

Psychological interventions should always be integrated in the treatment plan, because they reduce depressive symptoms and are not invasive.[14] Several models have been developed that target different elements of depression. For example, cognitive behavior therapy can effectively address depression-inducing cognitive styles (eg, catastrophizing) in patients whose cognitive and emotional function allows active engagement in therapy. Similarly, positive life review–based approaches (eg, dignity therapy) and meaning-oriented approaches (eg, meaning-centered psychotherapy) can promote a sense of purpose and decrease depressive symptoms and despair. Integrative medicine approaches (eg, music therapy) can decrease isolation and despair by promoting connectedness between the patient and family caregivers and can be provided throughout the continuum of care, including end of life.[15,16]

Assessment and management of anxiety

Although symptoms of anxiety are common and expected in serious and advanced illness, it is important to differentiate between symptoms of anxiety and anxiety disorders. Anxiety symptoms are a normal manifestation of fearful anticipation; for example, waiting for test results or waiting for a family meeting in which important medical decisions will be discussed. Transient anxiety can be adaptive and even help the patient and the family mobilize necessary energies while navigating the medical system and pursuing treatment options. When anxiety is not clinically significant, the level of arousal returns to baseline after the perceived threat or danger is controlled or neutralized, and the patient can continue functioning.

However, when anxiety becomes persistent and significantly interferes with psychosocial functioning, the presence of an anxiety disorder (generalized anxiety disorder, panic disorder) should be considered and assessed. Depending on the assessment method used, the prevalence of anxiety disorders in palliative care patients has been described between 10% and 30%.

Undertreated persistent anxiety causes a severe burden for the patient and family caregivers. It causes significant suffering, decreased trust in medical providers, a decreased ability to participate in medical decisions, and an increased interest in hastening death. Note that patients with poorly managed anxiety have also a decreased expectation that they will receive optimal symptom control at end of life.[13,17]

The clinical features of anxiety include physical, psychological, and cognitive symptoms:

Physical
- Diaphoresis
- Nausea
- Dizziness
- Tachycardia or tachypnea
- Palpitations
- Chest discomfort
- Gastrointestinal distress

Psychological
- Feeling edgy or unsettled
- Feeling irritable
- Feeling fearful and dreading the future

Cognitive
- Continual worrying
- Hypervigilance
- Difficulty integrating and processing information
- Rumination
- Catastrophizing

Medical conditions and medications can mimic, precipitate, or worsen anxiety. Poorly managed pain and symptoms, especially dyspnea, are common causes of anxiety. Corticosteroid treatment or stimulants can also cause or worsen anxiety. Psychosocial factors that create or worsen anxiety include uncertainty about the future, family conflict, financial concerns, and poor communication with medical providers. Fear of dying and fear of being in pain can also create severe anxiety.

Patients and family caregivers should be routinely screened for anxiety symptoms to ensure the prompt recognition of the development of an anxiety disorder. Brief screening tools (eg, the Patient Health Questionnaire for Anxiety and Depression) can be incorporated into routine visits. Additional assessment questions include:

- Do you ever feel you cannot stop worrying?
- Have you been feeling fearful or worried?
- Do you tend to always envision the worst-case scenario?
- Have people around you said you seem tense, edgy?
- Do you ever wake up in the middle of the night and start worrying?

As with depression, treatment choices for the management of anxiety depend on the patient's level of function, ability to engage in treatment, and prognosis. Psychological, behavioral, and integrative medicine approaches, if feasible, should always be considered to increase the patient's sense of control and personal agency. Cognitive behavior therapy can promote reality testing and coping by addressing cognitive distortions and maladaptive cognitive styles (ie, automatic negative thoughts and catastrophizing). Clinical hypnosis, relaxation, and mindfulness practices can decrease arousal and promote physical and mental relaxation and well-being.[18,19]

Pharmacologic treatment is chosen based on the patient's prognosis, treatment goals, and side effect profile. The presence of acute severe anxiety in advanced illness is a medical emergency and requires the use of benzodiazepines (eg, lorazepam or alprazolam). Anxiety in the context of neuropsychiatric syndromes (eg, terminal delirium) is generally managed with a neuroleptic. If the patient's life expectancy is greater than 2 to 3 months, first-line treatments include SSRI antidepressants (eg, escitalopram, citalopram, and sertraline) and SNRI antidepressants (eg, duloxetine and venlafaxine). Gabapentinoids (eg, gabapentin) are also frequently used.[13]

Coping with the grieving process during illness The grieving experienced by patients and family caregivers from the time of diagnosis throughout the illness trajectory is a normal and expected reaction to their past, present, and anticipated losses. Grieving occurs not only when the loss (ie, death) has occurred but is also triggered as this loss is feared and anticipated, and is commonly known as anticipatory grief. That is, patients grieve anticipating their own death and family caregivers grieve as they begin to imagine life without the patient. In addition, patients and caregivers grieve numerous progressive physical and psychosocial losses during illness (**Box 2**).

Providers should never make assumptions about what, why, and how individuals are grieving.

Because of cultural factors and personal grieving style, they may not appear overtly sad or despondent. The provider can support the grieving process by simply asking the patient and family caregivers how they are managing sadness and grief, showing openness, caring, and availability. This attitude can be reassuring and offer patients and family caregivers permission to talk about their grief, express their concerns, and receive psychoeducation about the grieving process.

The way people feel and express grief is deeply affected by their culture and personal history. However, it is important to avoid generalizations about what this means. It is more culturally and clinically appropriate to explore these aspects during the clinical encounter, allowing the patient and the family to educate the clinician about their experience and what they consider appropriate and important (**Table 2**). Ensuring that

Box 2
Examples of physical and psychosocial losses common in serious illness

Examples of physical losses for the patient

- Loss of body parts caused by surgery; for example, modified radical mastectomy
- Loss of function caused by adverse effects from treatment; for example, neuropathic pain, fatigue after chemotherapy
- Facial disfigurement after head and neck surgery
- Loss of physical comfort caused by pain and symptoms
- Progressive loss of independence

Examples of psychosocial losses for the patient and family caregivers

- Feeling that the body has betrayed them
- Progressive loss of spousal roles and intimacy caused by focus on caregiving tasks
- Loss of job, which can lead to loss of status, loss of income, loss of financial stability
- Loss of a sense of personal future and potential

Table 2
Cultural variations in the grieving process for patients and family caregivers

Aspects of Grieving	Cultural Variations
Private and public expression of grief	• How it is expected that grief will be expressed in the patient's culture? Through psychological manifestations (eg, crying, sadness) or through physical symptoms (eg, GI distress, pain)? • Is it considered appropriate in the culture to openly acknowledge and express the pain of grief; eg, crying in public, share personal distress with medical providers, ask for help in managing daily routines, request grief counseling?
Belief in an afterlife and communication with the deceased	• Is it normative in the culture to expect that communication with the decreased will continue through dreams, apparitions, or other form of communication? If these communications do not occur, is it assumed that the spirit of the deceased is angry?
Involvement of children and adolescents in grieving	• How is death explained to children in the culture? Are they integrated in community grieving and funerary practices or is it thought they should be protected by not participating?
What is considered normal and what is considered abnormal in grieving	• How quickly is the griever expected to adjust to the death of the loved one? How is it determined, in the culture, whether the grieving process has become unmanageable for the griever? • What interventions are acceptable or recommended in the culture to support grievers?
Relationship between meaning of death and grieving	• How is death understood and explained in the culture (eg, punishment, normal fact of life, necessary for accessing a better condition) • Does the construct of good or bad death exist in the culture? If so, what are the elements? How can these be incorporated in the care of the patient and the family?

Abbreviation: GI, gastrointestinal.

patients and family values during grieving are respected promotes trust with the provider and may be a protective factor for the development of complications.

Coping with the grieving process in bereavement Although the pain of losing a loved one may feel unbearable, most caregivers do, over time and with adequate social support, progressively integrate the pain of loss (**Table 3**) and continue engaging in life and relationships. Therefore, in a normal grieving process, the family caregiver slowly accepts the reality of the loss, slowly processes the pain of grief, and gradually finds a new way of existing in a world without the loved one.[20]

However, for some the grieving process becomes symbolically stuck, preventing them from processing the loss and adjusting. When this occurs, serious psychological and psychiatric complications can develop, most notably clinical depression and prolonged grief disorder (PGD).

Because the grieving process is unique for each individual, it is not always possible to predict how people will integrate the pain of losing a loved one and whether their grieving will become complicated. However, several factors have been identified that can be protective or increase risk in bereavement.[21] These factors are primarily related to the circumstances of the death, the personal psychological history of the family caregiver, the quality of the relationship with the patient during the illness, the experience of being a caregiver, and the quality of the relationship with the patient's treating team (**Box 3**).

Disenfranchised grief is an important risk factor. Any time someone openly grieves a loss that is not considered a major loss by their community or society, their grief may become disenfranchised. That is, they do not feel they have permission to express strong feelings openly, or it is expected that their reactions will subside in a very short time.

When the patient or family caregivers grieve losses that are not openly supported by society or the community, they are deprived of their opportunity to grieve openly and receive support. This situation can exacerbate the grieving process and present a risk factor for psychological and psychiatric complications, including depression, anxiety disorders, and suicidal ideation and behavior. For example, LGBTQ patients or family caregivers are at risk for disenfranchised grief in hospitals and clinics where providers make heteronormative assumptions or fail to acknowledge the relationship.[22–25] In essence, any individual facing discrimination and racism is at high risk for experiencing disenfranchised grief. However, patients and families may not openly share their challenges for fear that their concerns will not be heard, or that reporting will worsen the situation.

Table 3		
Expected manifestations of distress that improve over time in normal grief		
Physical	**Psychological**	**Cognitive**
Dizziness; nausea; heart palpitations; GI distress; anorexia; impact on cardiac, immune, and endocrine function	Anxiety, profound sadness, depressive symptoms, *transient* suicidal thoughts	Periods of impaired short-term memory, disorientation, decrease in concentration ability, *transient* perceptual disturbances (eg, auditory or visual hallucinations)

Data from Buckley T, Sunari D, Marshall A, et al. Physiological correlates of bereavement and the impact of bereavement interventions. Dialogues Clin Neurosc 2012;14(2):129–39; and Shear MK, Skritskaya NA. Bereavement and anxiety. Curr Psychiatry Rep 2012;14(3):169–75.

Box 3
Risk factors for psychiatric complications in bereavement

Quality of the relationship with the patient during illness
- High levels of ambivalence
- High levels of dependence

Psychological and psychiatric history of the bereaved family caregiver
- Prior psychiatric illness
- Lack of social support
- History of stressful life events
- Pessimistic attitude

Relationship with medical providers and the medical system during illness
- Poor communication with providers
- Conflict about treatment decisions
- Feeling that death was unexpected
- Disenfranchised grief

Quality of the caregiving experience during the patient's illness
- Feeling unprepared to deal with aspects of caregiving; for example, administer medications, wound care

Pain and symptom management
- Witnessing patient suffering caused by inadequate pain and symptom management

---

Awareness of risk factors is especially important for primary care providers, who can represent an important resource for bereaved family members. In many cases, they have been involved in the patient's care and are, therefore, aware of the challenges faced during the period of illness. The bereaved family member often remains under the provider's care. Every clinical encounter offers the provider an opportunity to assess the intensity of the grieving process and recognize the need to recommend bereavement support, including psychological intervention and even pharmacologic intervention to manage depression.

Bereavement research has also identified protective factors that have been associated with a smoother grieving process for bereaved family caregivers:

- Hospice care
- Social support
- Receiving adequate education and training to perform the tasks of caregiving for the loved one
- Feeling prepared for the death of the loved one

Psychiatric Complications in Bereavement: Bereavement-Related Depression and Prolonged Grief Disorder

Grieving processes in bereavement may not proceed smoothly. Although the expression of grief should never be pathologized, the development of psychiatric complications should never be discounted, normalized, or approached with nonspecific support.

Bereavement-related depression

Bereavement research has shown that grievers can develop clinical depression in the context of bereavement. Although depressive symptoms are common in grieving, grief and depression are 2 separate and distinct constructs, with different clinical features (see **Box 1**). Bereaved family members can develop depression during the illness of the loved one or in the aftermath of the death. In some cases, a depressed family caregiver may have remained undiagnosed during illness, so it is not always possible to determine a precise timeline for the development of depression. However, the key point is that depression should not be normalized as part of the grieving process.

Prolonged grief disorder

For almost 2 decades, researchers have agreed that the grieving process can become unmanageable and pathologic. The griever continues to experience severe and disabling symptoms on a daily basis, for a prolonged period of time, without any indication that adaptation is occurring.

Complicated grief and PGD are terms used for several years to describe pathologic grieving in bereavement. In an effort to facilitate recognition of pathologic grieving as a real and distinct disorder, different diagnostic criteria have been proposed because of a lack of agreement in terminology and conceptualization of pathologic grieving.[26]

However, in a recent development, PGD will be included in the International Classification of Diseases, 11th Revision (ICD-11). As a pathologic grieving process, it is recognized as a diagnostic entity different from normal grieving with specific criteria and applicability in the clinical setting.[27,28]

The main criteria are:

- Persistent and pervasive longing for the loved one
- Persistent and pervasive preoccupation with the loved one

In addition, the griever experiences intense emotional pain (ie, difficulty accepting the death, emotional numbness, difficulty engaging with social activities, inability to experience positive mood) that persists for at least 6 months after the death and causes severe impairment in functioning.

PGD is different from major depression, generalized anxiety disorder, or posttraumatic stress disorder. It describes a situation in which the griever continues to experience grief that remains severe and persistent, causing disabling and unremitting suffering.[29]

Psychological interventions are the most effective treatment approaches for pathologic grieving. In particular, modalities that include exposure to the memory of the loved one and target traumatic memories are effective in improving pathologic grieving.[30,31] Ongoing trials are evaluating the efficacy of grief-specific cognitive behavior therapy that specifically targets PGD.[32] Although antidepressants can be considered to address co-occurring depressive symptoms, they do not seem to be effective in relieving grief symptoms.[33] In addition, cultural aspects of grieving should always be carefully considered before diagnosing PGD, because the severity and length of the distress may be within cultural and social norms.

REFERENCES

1. Centor RM. To be a great physician, you must understand the whole story. MedGenMed 2007;9(1):59.
2. Payne R. Culturally relevant palliative care. Clin Geriatr Med 2015;31:271–9.
3. Tinetti M, Esterson J, Ferris R, et al. Patient priority-directed decision making and care for older adults with multiple chronic conditions. Clin Geriatr Med 2016; 32(2):261–75.
4. Johnson KS. Racial and ethnic disparities in palliative care. J Palliat Med 2013; 16(11):1329–34.

5. Lisy K, Peters MDJ, Schofield P, et al. Experiences and unmet needs of lesbians, gay, and bisexual people with cancer care: a systematic review and meta-synthesis. Psychooncology 2018;27(6):1480–9.

6. Baughman A, Clark MA, Boehmer U. Experiences and concerns of lesbian, gay, or bisexual survivors of colorectal cancer. Oncol Nurs Forum 2017;44(3):350–7.

7. Bristowe K, Hodson M, Wee B, et al. Recommendations to reduce inequalities for LGBT people facing advanced illness: ACCESSCare national qualitative interview study. Palliat Med 2018;32(1):23–35.

8. Badr H, Acitelli LK. Re-thinking dyadic coping in the context of chronic illness. Curr Opin Psychol 2017;13:44–8.

9. Kent EE, Rowland JH, Northouse L, et al. Caring for caregivers and patients: research and clinical priorities for informal cancer caregiving. Cancer 2016; 122(3):1987–95.

10. Turaga KK, Malafa MP, Jacobsen PB, et al. Suicide in patients with pancreatic cancer. Cancer 2011;117(3):642–7.

11. Yohannes AM, Alexopoulos GS. Depression and anxiety in patients with COPD. Eur Respir Rev 2014;23:345–9.

12. Pessin H, Breitbart WS. Suicide. In: Holland JC, Breitbart WS, Jacobsen PB, et al, editors. Psycho-oncology. 3rd edition. New York: Oxford; 2015.

13. Marks S, Heinrich T. Assessing and treating depression in palliative care patients. Curr Psychiatry 2013;12(8):35–40.

14. Farah WH, Alsawas M, Mainou M, et al. Non-pharmacological treatment of depression: a systematic review and evidence map. Evid Based Med 2016; 21(6):214–21.

15. Breitbart WS, Poppito SR. Individual meaning centered psychotherapy for patients with advanced cancer: a treatment manual. New York: Oxford University Press; 2014.

16. Bradt J, Dileo C, Magill L, et al. Music interventions for improving psychological and physical outcomes in cancer patients. Cochrane Database Syst Rev 2011;(8):CD006911.

17. Spencer R, Nillson M, Wright A, et al. Anxiety disorders in advanced cancer patients: correlates and predictors of end-of-life outcomes. Cancer 2010;116: 1810–9.

18. Montgomery GH, Schnur JB, Kravits K. Hypnosis for cancer care: over 200 years young. CA Cancer J Clin 2013;63:31–44.

19. Brugnoli MP. Clinical hypnosis for palliative care in severe chronic disease; a review and the procedures for relieving physical, psychological, and spiritual symptoms. Ann Palliat Med 2016;5(4):280–97.

20. Worden JW. Grief counseling and grief therapy. New York: Springer; 2009.

21. Thomas K, Hudson P, Trauer T, et al. Risk factors for developing prolonged grief during bereavement in family carers of cancer patients in palliative care: a longitudinal study. J Pain Symptom Manage 2014;47(3):531–41.

22. Jenkins CL, Edminson A, Averett P, et al. Older lesbians and bereavement: experiencing the loss of a partner. J Gerontol Soc Work 2014;57(2–4):273–87.

23. Fenge LA. Developing understanding of same sex partner bereavement for older lesbians and gay people: implications for social work practice. J Gerontol Soc Work 2014;57(2–4):288–304.

24. McNutt B, Oksana Y. Disenfranchised grief among lesbian and gay bereaved individuals. J LGBT Issues Couns 2013;7(1):87–116.

25. Bristowe K, Marshall S, Harding R. The bereavement experiences of lesbian, gay, bisexual and/or trans* people who have lost a partner A systematic review, thematic synthesis and modelling of the literature. Palliat Med 2016;30(8):730–44.

26. Jordan AH, Litz BT. Prolonged grief disorder: diagnostic, assessment, and treatment considerations. Prof Psychol Res Pract 2014;45(3):180–7.

27. Killikelly C, Maercker A. Prolonged grief disorder for ICD-11: the primacy of clinical utility and international applicability. Eur J Psychotraumatol 2018;8(Suppl 6): 1476441.

28. Patel SR, Cole A, Little V, et al. Acceptability, feasibility and outcome of a screening programme for complicated grief in integrated primary and behavioural health care clinics. Fam Pract 2019;36(2):125–31.

29. Maciejewski PK, Maercker A, Boelen PA, et al. Prolonged grief disorder and persistent complex bereavement disorder, but not complicated grief, are one and the same diagnostic entity: an analysis of data from the Yale Bereavement Study. World Psychiatry 2016;15:266–75.

30. Shear MK. Complicated grief treatment: the theory, practice, and outcomes. Bereave Care 2010;29(3):10–4.

31. Bryant RA, Kenny L, Joscelyne A, et al. Treating prolonged grief disorder: a 2-year follow-up of a randomized controlled trial. J Clin Psychiatry 2017;78(9): 1363–8.

32. Rosner R, Rimane E, Vogel A, et al. treating prolonged grief disorder with prolonged grief-specific cognitive behavioral therapy: study protocol for a randomized controlled trial. Trials 2018;19:241.

33. Bui E. Pharmacological approaches to the treatment of complicated grief: rationale and a brief review of the literature. Dialogues Clin Neurosci 2012;14(2): 149–57.

Ethical and Legal Considerations in End-of-Life Care

Frank Chessa, PhD[a],*, Fernando Moreno, MD[b]

KEYWORDS

- Ethics • End of life • Surrogate • Advance care planning
- Physician-assisted suicide • Palliative care • Palliative sedation • Futility

KEY POINTS

- Adopting a care plan that affects the manner and timing of a patient's death is an important moral responsibility.
- The ethical permissibility of a care plan likely to result in a patient's death depends on 3 factors: the causal pathway by which death occurs, the patient's prognosis, and the patient's preferences for care.
- Best practice in advance care planning includes enhancing communication with patients early in the disease process, documenting these conversations, and assisting patients to complete advance directives and appoint a Power of Attorney for Health Care.

INTRODUCTION
The Role of Ethics in Health Care

In its most general formulation, ethics provides guidance about how to live. For example, ethical theories identify character traits that we should instill in ourselves and the actions we should perform. Ethical frameworks do not presume that there is a single correct way to live, but they do hold that it is possible to evaluate individuals and actions as ethically better or worse. Ethics also moves beyond the individual to describe the types of government and laws that should be in place for people living in communities. Ethics is a somewhat unique discipline in that it attempts to describe the way the world *should be*, rather than the way it *is*.

Health care ethics asks the traditional questions of ethics in the context of individuals' health behaviors, the provision of health care services, and the governmental

Disclosure: The authors have nothing to disclose.
[a] Maine Medical Center, Tufts University School of Medicine, 22 Bramhall Street, Portland, ME 04102, USA; [b] Department of Family Medicine and the Division of Palliative Medicine, Maine Medical Center, Hospice of Southern Maine, Tufts University School of Medicine, 180 US Route One, Scarborough, ME 04074, USA
* Corresponding author.
E-mail address: chessf@mmc.org

Prim Care Clin Office Pract 46 (2019) 387–398
https://doi.org/10.1016/j.pop.2019.05.005
0095-4543/19/© 2019 Elsevier Inc. All rights reserved.

structures that affect health and well-being. Clinical ethics, the focus of this article, is a further specialization that concentrates on the interaction of clinicians, patients, and families in the direct provision of care.

Clinical ethics went through a transformation in the 1960s. Before this period, medicine primarily relied on guidance developed within the profession of medicine. A central example is Thomas Percival's *Medical Ethics*, which was adapted into the American Medical Association's first Code of Ethical Conduct in 1847.[1] In the 1960s, rising distrust in authority led to the environmental and consumer advocacy movements. These same sentiments also resulted in pressure for medicine to be more accountable. The development of intensive care units (ICUs), ventilators, dialysis, and organ transplants in the 1960s provided additional motivation to revisit professional codes of ethics. The consensus ethical guidelines discussed in this article are the result of multidisciplinary work that has progressed in the intervening decades. They result from an amalgamation of influences, reflecting traditions in medicine that are millennia old, religious and philosophic viewpoints, as well as recent changes in how society views, for example, sexuality and reproduction. Clinical ethics is a dynamic field, changing in response to new technology, new knowledge, and developing societal expectations. Nonetheless, a foundational characteristic of clinical ethics is that it is a rational enterprise—it seeks to use the best available evidence and sound reasoning to reach conclusions.

Methodology in Clinical Ethics

In many clinical situations, the answer to an ethical question will be well settled, and the practitioner need only turn to appropriate resources (such as, one hopes, the present document) to learn the answer. In other circumstances, the uniqueness or complexity of a case requires the skillful application of a method to reach an ethically sound decision.

The most prominent method is the principles method, advocated by Beauchamp and Childress.[2] The principles method relies on the 4 familiar principles of bioethics: respect for patient autonomy, nonmaleficence, beneficence, and justice (**Table 1**).

An ethical question is generated in a particular clinical case when 2 or more of the principles conflict. Beauchamp and Childress recognize that some conflicts between principles are so common that we have settled on standard answers (eg, waiving informed consent to provide emergency life-saving treatment to a patient who lacks decision-making capacity). In situations without standard answers, Beauchamp and Childress recommend a process of "balancing." They hold that the principles are not hierarchical (that is, no principle is an automatic trump of another). Instead, practitioners must decide which principle is more important in the context of a particular case, and devise a plan that honors that principle. They hold that the balancing process is a rational process that includes articulating specific reasons in favor of the

Table 1 Ethical principles	
Beneficence	Act for the Benefit of Others
Nonmaleficence	One ought not inflict evil or harm
Respect for autonomy	Respect the right of persons "to hold views, to make choices and to take actions based on their values and beliefs"
Justice	The benefits, risks, and costs of health care should be distributed fairly

choice made, as well as other criteria. Beauchamp and Childress do not claim that every practitioner will land on the same answer; they believe that the moral landscape is so rich, and the questions so nuanced, that reasonable practitioners acting in good faith may still disagree. Nonetheless, they hold that the process weeds out common errors in moral reasoning and leads practitioners to better decisions. In some ways, the balancing method works best as a group exercise: reasons are publicly articulated and critiqued from a variety of perspectives; creative, iterative problem solving allows the group to refine a plan—for example, adding features to mitigate the moral harms that arise from appropriately overriding one principle in favor of another.

Several other methodologies have been suggested as preferable.

- *Four box*: Morally relevant facts are grouped in 4 domains: Medical Indications, Patient Preferences, Quality of Life, and Contextual Features.[3]
- *Ethics of care*: Focuses on relationships and power differentials, rather than a rights-based approach to the resolution of disputes. For example, attending to the emotional relationships among 2 sisters and their dying father may do more to resolve a dispute about life-sustaining treatment than would focusing on the patient's right to self-determination.[4]
- *Narrative ethics*: Seeks to uncover ethical considerations by imagining the narrative that each stakeholder tells about their role in the case. For example, does the patient see their impending death as the culmination of a rich life, or as an unfinished story, the second half of which will not be written?[5]
- *Virtue theory*: Resolving an ethical dispute is a matter of skill rather than an exercise in applying principles. Skills include the ability to discern morally relevant attitudes and emotions and to comport oneself (in words, actions, and emotional attitude) in a way that resolves moral tensions.[6]

From the authors' perspective, each of the methods highlights important features in the moral landscape. In its focus on communication, palliative medicine incorporates insights from these methods, for example, with attentiveness to power differentials, awareness of the self-image that stakeholders bring to a case, control over one's own choices, and nonverbal communication in family meetings.

EVALUATING THE PERMISSIBILITY OF TREATMENT PLANS NEAR THE END OF LIFE

In some circumstances, clinicians adopt a plan of care that is likely to result in the death of a patient. This is a weighty responsibility, but one that cannot be avoided. Sometimes the treatment plan will involve withdrawing interventions that are directly supporting life, for example, a ventilator. Other times, the plan will have a less certain outcome, for example, treating a patient who has advanced dementia and aspiration pneumonia with empiric antibiotics, oxygen, and morphine for dyspnea, rather than hospitalizing him. Patient and family desires may also vary. Some patients hope for a quick death whereas others hope to survive, even while they refuse treatments they perceive as overly burdensome. In this section, we answer the question: under what conditions is it ethically appropriate to adopt a plan of care that is likely to result in the death of a patient? The conditions are grouped into 3 categories: prognosis, causal pathway, and patient preferences.

Prognosis

The ethical principle of beneficence highlights the importance of promoting a patient's best interest. To this end, the patient's prognosis and quality of life with life-prolonging treatment should be compared with the prognosis and quality of life when life-sustaining treatment is limited. The basic idea is simple: it is morally suspect to limit life-prolonging treatment when such treatment would return the patient to a quality of life that he or she has heretofore found acceptable. By contrast, if the prognosis is poor even with life-prolonging treatment, a plan of care that focuses on comfort is ethically reasonable.

This simple formula can be difficult to apply, as there are 2 complicating factors. First, there is often significant uncertainty about prognosis,[7] with physicians tending to be overly optimistic about prognosis.[8] Physicians who form enduring relationships with patients over time, such as family physicians, tend to overestimate prognosis. These factors can create disagreement about which treatment pathway will promote a patient's best interest.

The second complicating factor involves balancing the practitioner's view of quality of life with that of the patient. Practitioners must maintain some objectivity about quality of life, otherwise it would make no sense to counsel a patient to stop drinking alcohol to excess after the patient claims that his or her quality of life is better with this practice. Similarly, if a patient does not seem to appreciate that a life-prolonging treatment option will provide an acceptable quality of life (a quality the patient has found acceptable in the past), it is ethically justified for the practitioner to delay a decision until the issue is explored. This is not a license to impose practitioner judgments about quality of life on a patient; it simply recognizes that promoting a patient's best interest is morally important, even though it is tempered by respect for patient autonomy.

Causal Pathway

It is difficult to overstate the importance of the distinction between killing a patient and allowing a patient to die. The distinction underlies the laws, regulations, and policies relevant to end-of-life care in the United States. In brief, when the appropriate conditions are met, allowing a patient to die is ethically and legally permissible in all jurisdictions in the United States. By contrast, killing a patient is not permissible. The reasons for mercy killing, pain relief, a patient's request—are irrelevant to its legal permissibility. Indeed there have been challenges to this position. Famously, James Rachels argued that the distinction between killing and letting die is not morally relevant.[9] He argued that the moral badness of a killing or a letting die does not reside in action (or inaction) leading to the patient's death. Instead, the badness is explained by other factors (for example, the agent's intention or the patient's loss of the opportunities afforded by a longer life). This view has been echoed in more recent publications supporting physician assistance in dying. Nonetheless, Rachel's view has not made significant inroads regarding mercy killing.

Withdrawing versus withholding

Withholding a life-sustaining treatment (LST) and withdrawing an LST are both considered to be forms of letting patients die of their underlying disease or condition. Historically, some argued that withdrawing a treatment is impermissible (because it requires an action and is therefore analogous to killing), even while withholding the same treatment would be permissible (because this merely is an omission of an action). This argument did not win the day, however. In particular cases, there may be practical reasons to prefer withdrawing to withholding (or vice versa), and so in particular cases one pathway may be morally preferable to the other. Nonetheless, there is nothing in the nature of withholding or withdrawing that differentiates their baseline moral status. Withholding and withdrawing LST are now usually combined under the general term "forgoing" LST.

Medical nutrition and hydration

A similar debate occurred around the status of medical nutrition and hydration (MN&H). In the Cruzan case, the US Supreme Court found that there is no fundamental moral difference between MN&H and other medical treatments, and thus it is permissible to forgo MN&H.[10] Although this decision reflects current law, the issue is often encountered in clinical practice. The idea of a loved one "starving to death" raises strong emotions, and it is usually apparent to family members whether or not a patient is receiving nutrition. In addition, some religious groups hold that MN&H has a special moral status. For example, guidance from the US Conference of Catholic Bishops holds that, in principle, it is obligatory to provide MN&H, even for patients with brain injuries that result in permanent unconsciousness. Catholic health care directives also recognize that MN&H can be burdensome for the dying patient, and so it may be forgone in that circumstance.[11] For these reasons, it is important to preemptively discuss plans for nutrition and hydration.

Physician-assisted suicide

Physician-assisted suicide (PAS) involves the patient taking an action that causes his or her own death. Proponents of PAS have sometimes challenged this way of thinking, arguing that the ultimate cause of death is a terminal illness, and the patient, in taking action, is only controlling the manner in which the illness takes his or her life. For this reason, proponents advocate renaming the practice "medical aid in dying." The national discussion about PAS is well publicized.[12] In states where it is legal, the cause of death is not suicide but rather the terminal illness.

It is beyond the scope of this article to provide a full discussion of the arguments for and against PAS. Suffice it to say that arguments against the practice take 2 general forms: (1) the claim that suicide is always wrong, regardless of any good consequences that might follow from the action; (2) the claim that the legalized practice of PAS has bad consequences for society, for example, eroding a general respect for life, or the potential for the economic or emotional coercion of patients into using the practice. Proponents of PAS underscore the importance of patient autonomy and offer counterarguments to the aforementioned points. The guidance provided for clinical practice is straightforward: physicians in states where the PAS is not legal should refrain from its practice; physicians in states where it is legal should educate themselves about the practice and make an informed decision about whether they wish to participate. If they choose to participate, they should do so in accordance with their state's regulations.

Voluntarily stopping of eating and drinking

Dying patients eventually cease eating and drinking as a consequence of the dying process. For certain disease processes, changes in oral intake can be anticipated. For example, patients with advanced dementia often develop dysphasia with the consequent aspiration and recurrent pneumonias. In these circumstances patients and families are encouraged to significantly reduce or avoid oral feedings. This stepwise decline in feeding tolerance is thought to reflect underlying physiologic changes whereby patients often have decreased appetites and desire for food and drink. There is a difference, however, between those who stop eating *because they are dying* and those who die *because they stop eating*. The term "voluntary stopping of eating and drinking" (VSEAD) refers to the intentional choice by an adult with capacity to stop all forms of oral intake with the goal of hastening the dying process. For some patients, VSEAD is regarded as an opportunity to preserve control at the end of one's life, especially given that PAS is illegal in most states. Although no laws prohibit VSEAD, there are ethical concerns. The right of adult patients to refuse MN&H is well established, but typically this is done in advanced illness or severe neurologic injury and, in addition, the gastric tube (or other mechanism) used to provide MN&H carries risks and burdens. However, patients can pursue VSEAD at any stage of illness, and indeed death may be due to dehydration rather than the underlying disease. VSEAD typically carries significant burdens (patients must suppress their thirst), which suggests the patient's intention is to cause death rather than avoid the burdens of taking nutrition and hydration. Despite concerns, VSEAD is generally regarded as ethically permissible for patients with an advanced diagnosis that is expected to result in death.

When patients in the advanced stages of illness stop eating and drinking, there are often few symptoms associated with this decrease in nutrition and fluid. Conversely, the body seems to have protective mechanisms such as the release of endorphins that provide relief. Administering MN&H often worsens symptoms such as congestion and edema. However, for patients physiologically able to tolerate fluid and nutrition, cessation of oral intake can produce uncomfortable symptoms such as thirst and hunger. These symptoms can be incredibly difficult to withstand because of the strong innate survival mechanisms to maintain fluid and electrolyte homeostasis. Patients will often automatically break their fast because of intolerable thirst, although hunger is often better tolerated. Ethical questions arise about whether a practitioner should help palliate symptoms, and the answer will often depend on the stage of illness, suffering associated with the illness, and the patient's informed and voluntary choice of VSEAD. It may be prudent to seek consultations with colleagues, ethicists, and palliative medicine specialists in these complex cases.

The double effect of pain medication

Many medical treatments have both good and bad effects. Chemotherapy carries the risks of neutropenia, infection, and death, even while it carries the hope of inducing a cancer remission and longer life. In a patient with respiratory compromise, opioids carry the risk of further respiratory depression and death (although the extent of the risk is debated), even while they relieve suffering from air hunger. The doctrine of double effect (DDE) has been used to identify the circumstances when the bad effect of an action can be tolerated in the attempt to achieve the good effect. A common formulation of DDE includes 4 criteria:

1. The act must not be intrinsically wrong
2. The agent intends only the good effect (although the bad effect may be foreseen)
3. The bad effect must not be the means of achieving the good effect
4. The good effect is more important than the bad effect

DDE is used in end-of-life care to explain why an action that superficially looks like an impermissible killing (administering opioids that, in turn, cause respiratory depression and death) is actually a permissible instance of allowing a patient to die. In short, the relief of suffering is intended, while the risk of death is foreseen but not intended. Furthermore, in the case of a patient who is already dying from an underlying condition, the relief from suffering is more important than a slightly longer life.

As a practical guide, pain medication that carries a risk of death should be titrated up in response to discomfort and held constant after the discomfort is ameliorated. The reason for increasing the dosage should be documented because this provides evidence that one's intention is palliation rather than killing. Clinicians should consider a family's perception of patient suffering when palliating symptoms.

Palliative sedation to unconsciousness
Some patients at the end of life have symptoms that are difficult to control despite aggressive efforts. For such patients, it may be reasonable to consider sedating to the level of unconsciousness for the purpose of controlling symptoms. Palliative sedation refers to the practice of inducing unconsciousness with the intention of relieving suffering. Medications such as midazolam and phenobarbital are used with the intention of rendering of a patient unconscious when suffering cannot be controlled by other means. Many patients receiving palliative care at the end of life will experience sedation as a side effect of many of the medications used. For example, opioids, benzodiazepines, and antipsychotics all have the potential to cause sedation. However, these medications are administered with the intention to treat specific symptoms such as pain or dyspnea and not to produce sedation per se. In palliative sedation, the goal is to provide sufficient medication to render a patient unconscious.

Ethical concerns arise because patients rendered unconscious are unable to eat or drink; therefore, some equate the practice with killing. However, most patients requiring palliative sedation are often in the advanced stages of the dying process whereby eating or drinking would not be expected anyway. Palliative sedation is ethically permissible under the following conditions:

1. Severe pain or other physical symptoms that are refractory to treatment
2. Patient is close to death, with do-not-resuscitate order in place
3. Careful consent from patient or surrogate[13]

Family physicians considering palliative sedation are advised to obtain a palliative care and/or ethics consultation.[14,15] Professional guidelines support the use of palliative sedation when severe and refractory physical symptoms exist; however, its use to control the relief of nonphysical symptoms (such as depression or existential despair) is ethically problematic.

Patient Preferences

The final criterion for the permissibility of a care plan that is likely to result in the death of the patient is whether the patient does, or would, consent to the plan. The Cruzan case established that patients have a right to refuse LSTs.[10] It also established that this right survives the loss of the patient's capacity to make a contemporaneous choice. When the patient cannot make a contemporaneous choice, the right is exercised by examining the available evidence about what the patient would have wanted. "Substituted judgment" is the legal term for the determination of what the patient would have wanted were she or he able to understand the current options.

First-person consent
A person who provides informed consent makes a voluntary, informed, and reasoned choice. A recommended set of practices to achieve this ideal includes the following:

1. Determination of decision-making capacity
2. Assessment of the voluntariness of the action
3. Disclosure of information, including diagnosis, prognosis, treatment options, and the risks, benefits, and burdens of each option
4. Practitioner recommendation (if appropriate)
5. Assessment of understanding (using the teach back method)
6. Reflection and choice
7. Legal authorization (oral or written, documented as appropriate)[2]

Decision-making capacity

A crucial task for family physicians is determining whether a patient has the capacity to make a decision. Capacity differs from legal competence, which is determined by a court of law. Grisso and colleagues[16] developed the standard criteria for capacity:

- Ability to communicate choices
- Ability to understand relevant information
- Ability to rationally manipulate information
- Ability to appreciate the situation and its consequences

Capacity determinations are indexed to a particular question. For example, a patient can have capacity to appoint a Power of Attorney, but may lack capacity to consent to cardiac surgery. Capacity also waxes and wanes, so a geriatric patient who is cognitively intact in the morning may come to lack capacity in the evening.[16]

Advance care planning

Sudore and Fried[17] offer a prominent critique of the traditional focus on advance directives and naming a Power of Attorney for Health Care (POAHC). They argue that advance directives are too general to provide specific clinical guidance and that POAHCs are often uneducated about both the patient's disease process and the patient's preferences. They suggest shifting focus from completing advance directives to enhancing conversations with patients and family early in the trajectory of the patient's disease process. Two programs that attempt to do just this are Respecting Choices and the Serious Illness Conversation Project (SCIP). Respecting Choices showed remarkable success in developing an advance care planning (ACP) system in LaCrosse, Wisconsin.[18]

From an ethical perspective, scripted ACP conversations seek to promote patient autonomy. Many patients have only a vague notion, if they have any at all, about what they want at the end of life. It is not until persons are educated about their disease and the medical options, and until they can reflect on the implications of the information for their lives, that they form specific preferences. ACP conversations are designed to prompt reflection to help patients form these preferences. Preferences elicited during these conversations are documented in advance directives and POLST (Physician Orders for Life-Sustaining Treatment) forms, which are maintained by the patient and incorporated into the medical record. Increasingly, electronic medical records include ACP notes, which are clinician documentation of ACP conversations, and which are easily retrievable at the point of care.

Advance directives

State laws and federal regulations recognize advance directives as a means to communicate patient choices after a patient has lost the capacity to make a contemporaneous choice. Most advance directive forms also allow for the appointment of a POAHC. There is variation among states in criteria for valid completion (eg, some states require notarization, others do not). State laws also vary on whether a POAHC can override the choice in an advance directive, or whether the advance directive overrides a POAHC. Advance directives are recommended for all adults—even healthy adults, whereby they could provide guidance in the event of an unexpected neurologic catastrophe. For this reason, advance directives are typically general, for example indicating only whether the patient wants LST in the event of terminal illness or permanent loss of consciousness. This general guidance may not be helpful when more nuanced clinical decisions are required.

Physician/medical orders for life-sustaining treatment

POLST forms are appropriate for persons approaching their last year of life. Because the disease trajectory is known, POLST forms are designed to include more specific clinical guidance. POLST forms contain sections on cardiopulmonary resuscitation (CPR) status, MN&H, and intensity of treatment. POLST forms are typically signed by a provider and by the patient or patient's legally authorized surrogate. POLST forms are designed to be "portable" physician orders, such that they constitute valid orders regardless of the institution or setting in which the patient is located. A few states enacted legislation that gave them this legal status. More commonly, however, POLST forms serve as prima facie evidence of a patient's preferences, and their use is considered best practice.

Surrogate decision making

Ethically, the role of a surrogate decision maker is to promote patient autonomy by identifying what the patient would want were the patient able to speak. State laws often identify this role for surrogates, even while granting surrogates the authority to make decisions largely untethered to the concern about what a patient would choose for him- or herself. Communication with surrogates should reinforce the role of "being the patient's voice," in contrast to the surrogate choosing based on his or her own values or hopes. An additional strategy involves collecting evidence about what a patient would want (from an advance directive, prior clinician documentation such as ACP notes, and other family members), and presenting this information to the legally authorized surrogate to aid in decision making. It should be noted that decision making is stressful for surrogates, often resulting in psychological symptoms months after the event.[19]

State laws vary on the identification of the legally authorized decision maker when no POAHC exists. Best practice is to promote autonomy by encouraging the patient to appoint a POAHC. Many states default to a family hierarchy if no POAHC exists (eg, moving from spouse, to adult child, to parent, to sibling). A problem with such hierarchies is that they may not reflect the patient's social reality; for example, a patient may be emotionally close with a cousin who lives nearby while not having had any recent contact with an estranged son. Navigating the relationship between the legally authorized surrogate and other family members can be challenging. This is another reason why appointing a POAHC is important.

In palliative medicine the patient and family unit are considered to be the focus of care. However, how we create and define our families is varied and not always apparent. Patients should always be asked to identify their close friends and family and to define their important relationships. Some laws and algorithms for determining the legally authorized surrogate are based on heterosexist assumptions. People who identify as part of the LGBTQ community are at risk of being ostracized or not included in the decision-making process. Many older LGBTQ patients have living memories of how these issues have played out, for example, during the early years of the HIV epidemic.

PEDIATRIC END-OF-LIFE CARE

Providing care to a dying child can be both meaningful and challenging. The locus of communication shifts away from the patient to one that includes the patient and the patient's parent(s). The ethical framework for pediatric decision making revolves around 2 issues.

Identification of the Adult Decision Maker

It can be challenging to determine who is legally authorized to make medical decisions for a child. State laws vary, and many laws were written when it was assumed that most children would have 2 parents who were married to each other. Societal openness to a wider variety of family relationships (eg, separated or divorced parents, remarriage, cohabitation, blended families) requires the investigation of family relationships to determine the appropriate adult decision maker(s), especially for crucial end-of-life decisions. Practitioners should also be sensitive to emancipated minor status, as well as state laws that may give some minors control over reproductive, sexual, mental health, and substance use treatment decisions.

A special ethical challenge occurs when parents refuse recommended care. When the refusal creates significant risk for the child, this is termed medical neglect and it must be reported to state authorities.[20] Parents have discretion in making medical decisions for children, for example, in refusing childhood vaccinations. Thus, practitioners should be open to offering reasonable alternative treatments if their initial recommendation is refused. Near the end of life, parents may request a sole focus on comfort care before practitioners consider that life-extending treatment options have been exhausted. These cases can be very challenging, and consultation with pediatric palliative specialists or clinical ethicists is encouraged.

Participation of the Child in Decisions

For adults, practitioners consider both a patient's best interest and the patient's preferences in making medical decisions. Because infants and very young children have not developed informed and reasoned preferences, it is inappropriate to use the substituted judgment standard. For infants and very young children, decision makers should consider only the best interest of the patient. (Older children and adult patients with severe, lifelong cognitive impairment fall into this same category of "not previously competent" patients.)

The American Academy of Pediatrics (AAP) recommends that children participate in their health care decisions commensurate with their development.[21] However, state laws vary on the role of children in medical decision making, with a significant number drawing a "bright line" at 18 years old, before which parents have sole decision-making authority. The divergence between professional guidelines and state law can produce ethical tensions. In addition, a perennial issue with the AAP approach is how to share authority between parents and children. Some argue that if parents and practitioners have the ultimate authority to override a child's decision, it is disingenuous to tell the child that he or she can make decisions for him- or herself.[22] Ethical challenges also present themselves as pediatric patients age into late adolescence and adulthood. Patients may continue to look to parents and practitioners for decision-making support, or may seek independence from these "authority figures." Clinicians may risk alienating parents as they begin to prioritize the autonomy of a young adult.

DISPUTE RESOLUTION

Many ethical conflicts can be resolved with effective communication. Frequently, conflicts are the result of unclear communication. For example, a patient with metastatic cancer may understand that the disease has spread yet be unaware of its incurable nature. Such a patient may pursue high-burden interventions if he or she believes the benefits include substantial life prolongation. However, when informed about the incurability of the disease, the patient may be more likely to focus on other areas of his or her life. Relationships, unfinished business, and personal growth may become priorities. Even when the medical facts are agreed on, intense emotions might drive conflict. It is important to identify and provide opportunity for families to explore such emotion. For example, conflicts about whether to provide MN&H may be based in the sadness many feel when they watch their loved ones lose the pleasures associated with living. It is crucial to focus on these underlying conflicts in order to better support families through such emotional journeys to achieve a strong therapeutic alliance.

Caring for Diverse Populations

Clinicians are not expected to have an understanding of all of the world's cultures, or all the cultural differences that arise from differences in religion, racial identity, and socioeconomic status, among others. However, openness to considering another's world view is crucial to delivering patient-centered care. Cultural competence includes understanding that patients are likely to be experiencing their illness through a paradigm different from one's own. A respectful curiosity can often help clinicians meet patients and families from different cultures at a mutual place of respect. Often there are creative ways to honor the ethical principles even when, at first glance, they seem to conflict with a patient's cultural beliefs. For example, rather than consider full disclosure mandatory, it is now standard to ask patients how much information they want, how active they want to be in decision making, and how active they wants their families to be. This is a way to honor patient autonomy in the context of a culture that prizes family decision making.

Futile Treatment

The ethical debate regarding futile care is long standing. Futility disputes arise when clinicians consider that LST is no longer benefiting and perhaps is harming the patient while the patient or patient's family insists on continuing LST. The term "moral distress" was developed to name the negative emotion of ICU staff who feel trapped by the family, their institution, and the law into providing treatments they consider are morally wrong.[23] Current consensus reserves the term futile care for the rare situations in which an intervention has no chance of achieving its physiologic goal (eg, CPR after prolonged asystole). In these situations, physicians may unilaterally forgo the intervention. The more usual dispute involves interventions that have some chance of achieving the goal sought by the patient or family (such as keeping a patient alive for an additional week), but clinicians believe the intervention is unethical for other reasons (such as causing suffering in a dying patient). Current best practice recommendations suggest a procedural approach to dispute resolution, including ethics and palliative care consultation.[24]

SUMMARY

The ethical permissibility of a care plan likely to result in a patient's death depends on 3 factors: the causal pathway by which death occurs, the patient's prognosis, and the patient's preferences for care. If a care plan involves letting a patient die of their disease or injury, the patient has a poor prognosis, and the patient favors, or would favor, the care plan, the care plan is ethically permissible. If a care plan does not meet one or more of these criteria, the care plan may be ethically problematic and additional steps, such as advice from colleagues or expert consultation, are warranted.

REFERENCES

1. Thomas Percival (1740-1804), codifier of medical ethics. JAMA 1965;194(12): 1319–20.

2. Beauchamp TL, Childress JF. Principles of biomedical ethics. 7th edition. New York (NY): Oxford University Press; 2015.

3. Jonsen AR, Siegler M, Winslade WJ. The four topics: case analysis in clinical ethics. In: Jecker NS, Jonsen AR, Pearlman RA, editors. Bioethics: an introduction to the history, methods and practice. 2nd edtion. Sudbury (MA): Jones and Bartlett; 2007. p. 164–70.

4. Held V. The ethics of care: personal, political, and global. New York (NY): Oxford University Press; 2006.

5. Newton AZ. Narrative ethics. Cambridge (MA): Harvard University Press; 1995.

6. Giblin MJ. Beyond principles: virtue ethics in hospice and palliative care. Am J Hosp Palliat Care 2002;19(4):235–9.

7. Yourman LC, Lee SJ, Schonberg MA, et al. Prognostic indices for older adults: a systematic review. JAMA 2012;307(2):182–92.

8. Christakis NA, Lamont EB. Extent and determinants of error in doctors' prognoses in terminally ill patients: prospective cohort study. BMJ 2000;320(7233):469–72.

9. Rachels J. Killing and letting die. In: Becker LC, Becker C, editors. Encyclopedia of ethics. 2nd edition; 2001. p. 947–50.

10. Cruzan v. Director, Missouri Department of Health, (88-1503), 497 U.S. 261 (1990).

11. US Conference of Catholic Bishops. Ethical and religious directives for Catholic health care services. Washington, DC: USCCB; 2009.

12. Vacco v. Quill, 521 U.S. 793 (1997). Gonzales v Oregon (formerly Ashcroft v. Oregon) U.S. 131 (2011).

13. Graeff AD, Dean M. Palliative sedation therapy in the last weeks of life: a literature review and recommendations for standards. J Palliat Med 2007;10(1):67–85.

14. Cassell EJ, Rich BA. Intractable end-of-life suffering and the ethics of palliative sedation. Pain Med 2010;11(3):435–8.

15. National Ethics Committee, Veterans Health Administration. The ethics of palliative sedation as a therapy of last resort. Am J Hosp Palliat Care 2007;23(6):483–91.

16. Grisso T, Grisso A, Appelbaum PS. Assessing competence to consent to treatment: a guide for physicians and other health professionals. New York (NY): Oxford University Press; 1998.

17. Sudore RL, Fried TR. Redefining the "planning" in advance care planning: preparing for end-of-life decision making. Ann Intern Med 2010;153(4):256–61.

18. Hammes BJ, Rooney BL, Gundrum JD. A comparative, retrospective, observational study of the prevalence, availability, and specificity of advance care plans in a county that implemented an advance care planning microsystem. J Am Geriatr Soc 2010;58(7):1249–55.

19. Wendler D, Rid A. Systematic review: the effect on surrogates of making treatment decisions for others. Ann Intern Med 2011;154(5):336–46.

20. Pietrantonio AM, Wright E, Gibson KN, et al. Mandatory reporting of child abuse and neglect: crafting a positive process for health professionals and caregivers. Child Abuse Negl 2013;37(2–3):102–9.

21. Katz AL, Webb SA, Committee on Bioethics. Informed consent in decision-making in pediatric practice. Pediatrics 2016;138(2):e20161484.

22. Klass P. When should children take part in medical decisions. New York Times 2016.

23. Curtis JR, Burt RA. Why are critical care clinicians so powerfully distressed by family demands for futile care? J Crit Care 2003;18(1):22–4.

24. Bosslet GT, Pope TM, Rubenfeld GD, et al. An official ATS/AACN/ACCP/ESICM/SCCM policy statement: responding to requests for potentially inappropriate treatments in intensive care units. Am J Respir Crit Care Med 2015;191(11):1318–30.

Cultural, Religious, and Spiritual Issues in Palliative Care

Sally E. Mathew-Geevarughese, DO*, Oscar Corzo, MD,
Elizabeth Figuracion, DO

KEYWORDS

• Palliative care • Religion • Spirituality • Culture • Interdisciplinary team

KEY POINTS

- Although religiosity and spirituality tend to be lumped together, spirituality appears to be a broader concept that can be shared without having a theistic set of beliefs.
- Religion is typically associated with an organized system of beliefs, rituals, and practices. Religious individuals may consider themselves spiritual, whereas the opposite may not always be true.
- Suffering is often viewed as a normal part of the life cycle and upholding a commitment to long-standing religious beliefs.
- Spiritual struggle is known to have distressing effects, including depression, lower tolerance to physical symptoms, including pain, as well as a negative impact on the will to live.
- There are multiple points of cultural diversity that can define the approach to medical care, such as the family unit, care of the elderly, view of physicians, and views on death.

INTRODUCTION

As primary care physicians, the issues of culture, spirituality, and religion are topics we consciously or subconsciously shy away from. We may not feel comfortable talking with patients about these issues or we may not feel that we are properly equipped to address them. You may wonder how do I even know when there are such issues that need to be addressed? If so, how do I approach it? What could I offer to them?

Current research confirms that health care providers feel inadequately prepared to address the spiritual concerns of their patients and that there is a strong need for ongoing education regarding these matters.[1]

Disclosure: The authors have nothing to disclose.
Palliative Care Department, Jamaica Hospital Medical Center, 8900 Van Wyck Expressway Suite 3D, Jamaica, NY 11418, USA
* Corresponding author.
E-mail address: smathew7@jhmc.org

Primary care physicians are at the frontlines, often the first point of contact for many people within the medical system. They have to manage chronically ill patients with life-limiting diagnoses who also have ongoing psychosocial needs. We hope this article will provide you with the resources needed to identify any cultural, spiritual, or religious needs your patients may have, and build confidence in your ability to care appropriately for these patients and their families.

WHAT IS SPIRITUALITY?

Spirituality is not synonymous with religion, and the two do not always have to be associated with each other. Many definitions of spirituality have emerged and there is no consensus, although it continues to evolve over time.[2]

Spirituality is described in the literature as a "subjective, all-encompassing aspect of well-being, which entails the way individuals experience connectedness and meaning to themselves, others, and their environment."[3,4] Although religiosity and spirituality tend to be lumped together in common discourse, spirituality appears to be a broader concept that can be shared among people without having a theistic set of beliefs.[4,5] Integral elements of the spiritual experience include the intrapersonal (meaning in one's own life), as well as interpersonal (connectedness with others, in particular loved ones), and finally natural interconnectedness (experience of the natural world/beliefs including theism).[5,6]

Here are some common themes that were developed by Unruh and colleagues[1] to help us better understand this concept:

1. Relationship to God, a spiritual being, a Higher Power or reality greater than self
2. Not of the self
3. Transcendence or connectedness unrelated to a belief in a higher being
4. Existential, not of the material world
5. Meaning and purpose in life
6. Life force of the person, integrating aspect of the person
7. Summative definitions that combines multiple themes

Chao and colleagues[1] studied the essence of spirituality in a sample of terminally ill Buddhist and Christian patients, in which they found 4 major themes:

1. Communion with self (self-identity, wholeness, inner peace)
2. Communion with others (love, reconciliation)
3. Communion with nature (inspiration, creativity)
4. Communion with a higher being (faithfulness, hope, gratitude)

It is powerful to consider this aspect of your patient, as these qualities constitute who this person is. As primary doctors we aim to learn about our patient as a whole and how they interpret, interact, and deal with the world. This will affect how they deal with and interact with you as their doctor and with their health care decision making.

WHAT IS THE DIFFERENCE BETWEEN SPIRITUALITY AND RELIGION?

Religion is typically associated with an organized system of beliefs, rituals, and practices. Those who are religious may consider themselves spiritual, whereas there are those who consider themselves spiritual but not religious. It is important to realize that religion may not be a part of a person's spirituality. Religion may provide a motivational and disciplined framework for spiritual growth. Its meaning is transmitted through doctrine and stories of the community. Spirituality is not institutionally bound;

it is concerned with discovery of meaning in the context of the level individual, and is concerned with self-directed spiritual growth.[2]

The concepts of spirituality and religion should be considered, as they impact health outcomes. Research suggests that both play a positive role in individuals coping with cancer and human immunodeficiency virus. Studies also show that, for patients with advanced cancer, spiritual well-being and a strong sense of meaning are important buffers against hopelessness, depression, and desire for hastened death.[1]

DO PATIENTS REALLY WANT US TO ADDRESS THESE ISSUES WITH THEM? WHY SHOULD WE CARE ABOUT IT?

The literature indicates that addressing spiritual issues are welcomed by many. A Gallup survey done in 1977 explored that spiritual beliefs in dying patients indicated that in addition to turning to family members (81%), close friends (61%), and clergy (36%) for support at the end of life, 30% would look to doctors for support. Others may be hesitant to bring this topic up to their doctors, as they do not want to burden busy professionals.[1]

In another Gallop poll conducted in January 2002, 50% of Americans identified as "religious" but 33% stated they are "spiritual but not religious."[7] In 2017, 37% of Americans perceived themselves to be highly religious, whereas another 30% identified as moderately religious.[8] A slim majority of Americans (55%) believe that religion can answer most problems.[9] Although most of those polled in these studies identify with a Christian denomination, this belief provides much-needed insight into potential conflicts that can arise during medical care.

Additional studies observe religious and spiritual interplay with medical decision making in people with advanced cancer diagnoses. In the federally funded Coping with Cancer Study, 230 people with advanced cancer diagnoses and a prognosis of less than 1 year were interviewed about their spiritual needs, religiosity, quality of life, and treatment preferences.[10] Even though 68% of participants felt religion was very important and 20% felt it was somewhat important to them, close to half (47%) felt their spiritual needs were met minimally or not at all by their religious community. A large percentage (72%) felt minimal or no support from their medical teams. Having this support from their religious and medical community was associated with a better quality of life.[10] A higher level of religiousness also was associated with wanting aggressive measures to prolong life.[10]

Several case reports take a closer look at the religious impact on medical decision making with various ethnic groups. With religion involved, Latino patients and families were more hesitant to deescalate care, as they viewed this equal to killing their loved one, whereas Cambodian patients were able to distinguish between the two.[11] Both cohorts greatly valued input from their physician and if their loved one was likely to have poor quality of life, they would be more open to the idea of deescalating care. The idea of suffering, however, does not always readily lead to deescalation of care.

Suffering is often viewed as a normal part of the life cycle and upholding a commitment to long-standing religious beliefs. Inability to recognize this, however, can lead to the feeling of being unsupported in their care. Sickness and the associated suffering can be seen as a test or as punishment for a sin that was committed. Religious coping in the form of prayer, meditation, and religious study is practiced by many people to help them approach and adjust to their illness.[12] In a study conducted at Duke University Medical Center with 150 patients with advanced cancer, 78% wanted their religious community to support their spiritual needs but 66% also wanted support from their medical team.[12]

Many patients, even those who do not identify with a formal religious organization, want their physicians to ask about their spiritual health.[12] Spirituality allows a person to experience a transcendent meaning in life. This can be expressed not only as a relationship with God, but often about nature, art, music, family, or community, whatever beliefs and values provide a sense of meaning and purpose in life. Most people identify at least one spiritual need and appreciate the opportunity to pray with someone.[12] A significant number of patients (85%) felt the attention to this aspect of their care would improve their overall satisfaction with care.[12] Unfortunately, many studies show that spiritual needs are met minimally or not at all, correlating with lower satisfaction with care, lower quality of life, higher rates of depression, and higher costs of medical care.[13]

It may seem daunting that the responsibility of dealing with the spiritual concerns of patients is something primary care doctors must consider in the limited amount of time they have with patients. However, it is possible, and primary care doctors ought to be familiar with how to approach these issues. Hopefully you can find comfort in knowing that your patients would appreciate this kind of conversation with you. It adds another layer of trust and strengthens the patient-physician relationship.

EXISTENTIAL SUFFERING/SPIRITUAL PAIN

Spiritual concerns are a common element of the experience of illness. As such, spiritual struggle is known to have distressing effects on the afflicted individual, including depression, lower tolerance to physical symptoms including pain, as well as a negative impact on the will to live. Conversely, cultivation of spiritual well-being during illness is known to protect an individual's sense of self and connectedness, which has a beneficial impact on those concerns.[3] A study of 57 patients with cancer demonstrated that 96% of these patients experienced spiritual pain at some point in their lives, and 61% reported experiencing such struggle at time of interview.[3] Of these patients experiencing spiritual pain, 48% expressed intrapersonal pain, 38% religious spiritual pain, and 13% interpersonal spiritual pain, highlighting the prevalence of this aspect of suffering and the beneficial impact of proper assessment and intervention.[6]

Key spiritual concerns in patients at end of life involve, as broadly classified by Chaplain Dick Millspaugh,[14] issues of purpose and meaning, as well as death/finitude and the self, and are listed in **Table 1**. Issues of purpose and meaning tend to appear as functional capabilities decline and individuals are no longer able to maintain their routine or lifelong roles. Death/finitude issues arise as individuals are forced to come in imminent contact with their own mortality and experience a loss of their sense of control. As the individual loses purpose, meaning, and control, in the setting of end of life, the individual also experiences a greatly diminished sense of who they are in relation to themselves, others, and their environment. Reaching a clear understanding of the spiritual pain issues at play is essential to the development of a compassionate response and a spiritual care plan.[14]

Paramount among the immediate responses available to the practitioner is the concept of "compassionate presence."[6] Although it does not change an individual's medical/physical situation or prognosis, the simple act of acknowledging and being witness to an individual's suffering is of great healing value.[6] It inspires a multitude of spiritual aspects, including the capacity to be present in the world, to experience emotions, to connect with others, and to look to the future to formulate goals. The reality of what the individual is going through must be acknowledged, and practitioners must be willing to be with and suffer alongside as opposed to abstractly putting

Table 1		
Key spiritual concerns in serious illness and associated expressions		
Concerns of Purpose and Meaning	Concerns of Death/Finitude	Concerns of Self
Hopelessness • "There is nothing left for me to live for" Purposelessness • "I feel useless" Meaninglessness • "My life is meaningless" Loss of meaningful relationships • "No one comes by anymore" Loss of religious perspective • "God has abandoned me"	Imminent mortality • "Life is being cut short" Secondhand experience of finitude • Recounting death of friends/relatives Loss of control • "I can no longer live my life the way I want to"	Loss of the self (emotionally, spiritually, religiously, physically, or in the context of a relationship) • "I am not the person I used to be," "I no longer know who I am" Awareness of diminished sense of self • "My illness took everything away from me"

themselves in the situation at hand. The concept of pain as currently defined by the International Association for the Study of Pain describes it as experienced by humans in a nociceptive fashion: "pain is an unpleasant sensory and emotional experience associated with actual or potential tissue damage, or described in terms of such damage."[6] This has lent itself to dichotomizing pain into its physical and nonphysical components (psychological, spiritual, religious concerns). Although the importance of properly evaluating and treating physical pain is essential for comfort, it is important to understand that physical, psychological, and spiritual pain are interconnected, although separate, entities.[6]

The experience of spirituality, and thus potential areas for distress, are often described in terms of intrapersonal (related to an individual's view of the self), interpersonal (connections with other human beings), and interconnectedness with the environment and nature (which also can describe aspects of religion).[5,6] Intrapersonal spiritual pain involves a variety of spiritual distress domains, including despair, feelings of loss (eg, of the self, of control, of meaning), regrets, helplessness, and dread of impending mortality. The interpersonal spiritual pain domains include brokenness, alienation, and guilt. Interconnectedness/religion concerns feature separation from a faith community and abandonment by God.[3,6] This classification is described in **Fig. 1**.

When organized in this fashion, a few correlations of practical importance have been noted in the literature. Notably, patients older than 50 tend to experience less spiritual pain as part of the dying process than younger patients.[3] Younger patients with the promise of a fuller, longer life ahead of them tend to experience more spiritual distress, particularly in terms of despair, brokenness, helplessness, and meaninglessness.[3] Perhaps as a result, younger patients also tend to continue to receive aggressive medical treatment at end of life. Importantly, physical pain is another strong influencer of spiritual struggle, in much the same way. Further associations with spiritual distress include depression, which serves to worsen symptoms. Conversely, sustaining the spiritual aspect of patient care is associated with improved physical and psychological well-being.[3]

THE PRIMARY CARE DOCTOR CAN PROVIDE SPIRITUAL CARE: YES IT'S TRUE!

The interdisciplinary team shares the responsibility of assessing and addressing the spiritual needs of patients and families. This is not the sole responsibility of the

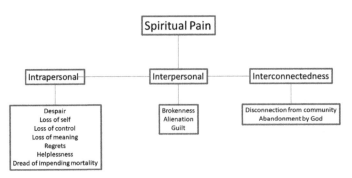

Fig. 1. Threefold model of spiritual pain with associated distress domains.

chaplain, clergy, or other designated professionals. The following issues were identified as barriers in a study of physicians with regard to providing spiritual care:

1. Marginalization and devaluation of psychosocial and spiritual care during medical training
2. Lack of safe and supportive environment in which to discuss issues of loss and death
3. Time demands and busy clinical schedules
4. Lack of training and skills-building in discussing existential issues with patients[1]

Health care providers cannot assume that all patients have spiritual needs that require constant attention, or that they will always look to health care professionals to help meet these needs. The health care team should evaluate to what extent the patient would like the team to be involved in addressing those issues. It is up to the clinician's own comfort level with providing spiritual care that also dictates their involvement. It has been suggested that providing good spiritual care depends on the clinician's awareness of a spiritual dimension in their life, honed communication skills, ability to establish a trusting relationship with patients, and to draw on their own life experience and maturity.[1]

HOW DO I BRING IT UP? SPIRITUAL ASSESSMENT

Spiritual screening serves as a basic survey of the patient's broad attitude toward spirituality and religion and also helps determine the level and immediacy of further spiritual care needs. This initial survey can be performed by the physician as well as a physician extender in the care team and is limited to general questions, such as "Is spirituality or religion an important aspect in your life?" and "How well are these sources of strength serving you at this time?"[4] Obvious signs of distress in response to this questions would invite prompt referral to a board-certified chaplain for a full assessment and development of a spiritual care plan.[4]

Spiritual history-taking is a more involved process that aims to better understand the patient's spiritual needs and current resources. The goals of the spiritual history include giving an opportunity for patients to share their spiritual/religious beliefs and values, define spiritual goals, look for spiritual distress elements, as well as elements of strength, provide compassionate care, and identify patients requiring more resources or a deeper assessment from a chaplain.[4] Various tools for spiritual history-taking are available including FICA, HOPE, and Open invite, as described later in this article.

To be an effective spiritual care provider, it is important to look inwardly to gauge the provider's own level of experience as a guide for relating to the patient. It is also useful to understand some of common spiritual concerns expressed by patients. Finally, the provider must be able to formulate a compassionate response that is consistent with the patient's spiritual values and belief systems.

By doing this, the practitioner gains perspective as related to their own suffering, which can prove of great value at creating a collaborative relationship with the patient:

- What do I know about being close to my own death?
- When have I lost significant relationships (to others, to God) in my life?
- How about losing the sense of the self?
- Have I ever lost a sense of purpose or meaning in my life?
- What helped and what did not?
- Can I even become close to knowing anything at all about what the other person is going through?
- Do I have any business offering solutions?[4,14]

Consider taking a spiritual assessment and offering spiritual support to be similar to taking a social history, and empathizing after delivering a negative diagnosis, or when the patient shares some bad news. Addressing spiritual concerns is another way we can understand and support patients throughout their experience of illness.[2]

WHAT ARE THE TOOLS?

There are some tools that can be used in your time-sensitive encounters with the patient. The goal is to engage the patient in open-ended questions to explore their spiritual concerns.

1. FICA Spirituality Tool: This is an acronym with a series of questions to elicit patient spirituality and its potential effect on health care.[2,15]

F	Faith and beliefs	Asking whether they have any spiritual beliefs or what gives their life meaning
I	Importance	Asking how these beliefs influence the way they take care of themselves
C	Community	Asking whether they are part of a religious or spiritual community
A	Address in Care	Asking how to address these issues as their provider

2. HOPE Tool: This addresses general concepts of hope, whether patients belong to an organized religion, their personal spirituality practices, and what effect their spirituality may have on medical care and end-of-life decisions.[2]
   H: Sources of hope
   O: Organized religion
   P: Personal spirituality and practices
   E: Effects on medical care and end-of-life issues[2]
3. Open Invite Tool: This is a patient-focused approach to encouraging an open spiritual dialogue. It reminds the physician that his or her role is to *open the door* to conversation and *invite*, never require, patients to discuss their needs. Preaching or prescribing spiritual practices is generally beyond the proper bounds of the physician-patient relationship. This tool allows the physician to broach the topic of spirituality. Questions are similar to those of the FICA and HOPE tool, or can

be customized. The key to this approach is to use questions and language that are natural and conversational while being respectful and nonthreatening.[2]

Examples include the following:

- May I ask if you have a faith or religion?
- Do you have a spiritual or religious preference?
- How does your spirituality or faith preference affect the health care decisions you make?
- Is there a way our team can provide you support with your spiritual or religious beliefs?[2]

ROLE OF CHAPLAIN/PASTORAL CARE REFERRAL

The mainstay of the approach to patient care in both primary and palliative care is the interdisciplinary team. The chaplain is an important member of this team as a professional who primarily focuses on the spiritual aspects of the patient. The chaplain can be a great resource when you as the physician may not be able to take the conversation further.

The ability to recognize spiritual distress in patients who question the meaning of life, are angry with God, ask where God is while they are suffering, and lose a sense of purpose and self-meaning is often a necessary first step to their individual journey through serious illness.[12] In a study conducted by chaplains at Calvary Hospital, nearly half of the patients described their pain in relation to an emotional state, such as feeling despair, loss, anxiety or regret, whereas 38% felt abandoned by God or without a faith community. Thirteen percent described being disconnected with their family members. Moreover, one-third of the patients described their pain physically as a "deep ache in their heart," an "explosion in their body," or "all over physical pain."[6]

In recent years, the chaplain has become a vital member of the health care team with a considerable expansion of responsibilities beyond administering prayers and rites. They are specially trained with a focus in addressing and providing spiritual support regardless of the patient's faith background. A specific health care institution, such as a hospital or hospice program or hospice house, usually employs chaplains. They can also be sponsored by a spiritual or religious denomination that actively supports the presence and work of chaplains in a given health care setting.[16]

Chaplains set an agenda for pastoral care that is committed to providing spiritual care to patients, family/friends, and staff. They are integral to facilitating communication and conflict resolution.[16]

The different expressions of spiritual care provided by the chaplain include the following:

1. Presence: active and empathetic listening.
2. Prayer: a broad spectrum of spiritual practice, including traditional liturgy, meditation, songs, guided imagery, and other.
3. Ritual: facilitating religious ceremonies and designing contemporary spiritual ceremonies incorporated into blessings, holiday worship and observance, and memorial services and funerals.
4. Learning texts as spiritual resources: traditional scriptures such as the Bible, Torah, Koran, Book of Buddha, and others, as well as contemporary prose and poetry. This often leads to theological reflection or more general "spiritual work" that a chaplain can help facilitate.
5. Advocacy: facilitating communication with all staff members, referring to other health care professionals and complementary spiritual therapies including music, art, relaxation training, guided imagery, and healing touch.[16]

AFTER THE SPIRITUAL ASSESSMENT IS COMPLETE, HOW CAN YOU INCORPORATE THESE RESULTS INTO YOUR PRACTICE?

The most basic, and sometimes the most difficult, thing we can do as physicians is to listen compassionately. Regardless of whether patients are devout in their spiritual traditions, their beliefs are important to them. By listening, we are showing our patients that we care and validate the importance of this aspect of their lives. Empathic listening may be all the support the patient needs.[2]

You can document the patient's spiritual perspective, background, impact on medical care, and openness to the topic. This may be helpful to refer to when re-addressing these concerns in the future or during times of crisis when sources of comfort and meaning become crucial. Documenting this can also meet hospital regulatory requirements for conducting a spiritual assessment.[2]

Physicians can incorporate this information by considering how different traditions and practices may affect medical practice. For example, Jehovah's witnesses usually refuse blood transfusions, whereas Muslim and Hindu women may decline sensitive physical examinations by male physicians. Staunch believers of faith healing will shy away from traditional medical care and hope for a miracle.[2]

Assessing spirituality can be a source of reinforcement the physician can give to his or her patient, especially if their practices are positive coping behaviors. This can include asking "do you have spiritual practices such as praying, meditating, listening to music, reading sacred text, that you find helpful or comforting?" Discussing these topics may allow us to learn about resources the patient can connect with if the patient is part of a faith-based community, including a home visitation program, food pantry, and health screening, for example. You may offer to contact their spiritual community to help mobilize these resources with the patient's permission.[2]

SHOULD I PRAY WITH MY PATIENT?

You may find yourself in a situation in which a patient asks you to pray with him or her. There is no right or wrong answer to this question, although the overarching concern is the comfort level of the practitioner. For example, if there is a shared faith tradition and level of religiosity, a physician-led prayer can further solidify the physician-patient relationship. If the physician is uncomfortable with praying, the physician can ask the patient to lead the prayer while remaining present during that experience. If the patient insists that a member or the medical team lead in prayer, the physician can set a time to return with the chaplain. It is imperative to recognize that prayer is not the goal of a thorough spiritual assessment, and physicians should not attempt to get patients to agree with them on specific faith issues.[2]

Other forms of response, mainly the expression of empathy and the continued listening to the patient's spiritual agenda, should be implemented with an awareness of the cultural and faith perspectives of the patient in mind. Care must be taken to maintain boundaries; to maintain a compassionate presence, the practitioner giving spiritual care should think of himself or herself as suffering with the patient as opposed to suffering for the patient. This is because although the practitioner may or may not have extensive secondhand experience with end-of-life concerns, most have not directly experienced what the patient is going through. It is similarly of primary importance for practitioners to avoid proselytizing or pressing their own beliefs on the patient: even if well-intentioned, it is an act made on behalf of the proponent rather than the patient and is thus inappropriate. It also represents a breach of trust, as the proponent would have been clearly aware of the patient's spiritual agenda.[4,5]

Atheism

Given the significant presence of religion in US culture, careful consideration should be extended to the spiritual care of patients who have no theistic belief system. As such, atheists represent a particular group not often described in the literature. Although spirituality in individuals (including atheists) can be understood within the context of the intrapersonal, the interpersonal, and the connection to nature/environment, atheists do not associate any of these connections to Gods, devils, souls, or other supernatural entities. Moreover, atheists express strong preferences toward communication and evidence-based interventions. Particular attention should be paid to respecting the terminology proposed by the patient. Many consider the term "atheist" objectionable, and prefer "freethinkers," skeptics," or "secular humanists." Similarly, the term "spiritual" is also problematic for these patients, and care should be taken to avoid the term during discussion.[4]

The components of a "good death" as described in a survey study of atheist preferences include the following:

1. Comfort: including pain and symptom relief using scientific, evidence-based measures.
2. Control over the dying process: distaste for futile care, desire to not be a burden to family, and queries about physician-assisted suicide.
3. Autonomy: including respect for nontheistic beliefs, no proselytizing, and no religious references.
4. Intrapersonal spirituality: reflection and rest, alone. Consideration for organ donation/donation of body to science.
5. Interpersonal spirituality: spending time with friends and family privately. Planning culturally appropriate memorial services.
6. Natural connectedness: time outside and with pets.[4]

Although providers with a strong religious background may find interaction with these patients challenging, and even unsettling, it is again important to realize that a religious background is not a requirement for having spiritual needs.[4]

Cultural Aspects of Care

Just as spirituality and religiosity are closely intertwined in the core aspects of an individual, so is the interplay of culture in medical decision making. The level of sensitivity required when approaching the cultural aspects of care mirrors the approach previously laid out in this article.

As the world's melting pot, America has embraced a continuously fluctuating cultural landscape. Many individuals and their families come to this country with hopes of gaining access to the latest innovations in medical science and, often times, a second chance at life. Building rapport and engaging in goals of care discussions can be a daunting task, especially if cultural influences in medical decision making are not considered.

HOW IS CULTURE DEFINED?

Culture can be defined as the set of shared attitudes, values, goals, and practices that characterizes an institution or organization.[17] The elements of culture include language, customs, rituals, spirituality and religion, government, and societal organization. Furthermore, how individuals approach their medical care is often influenced by their previous interactions with health care and input from their community.

HOW DO DIFFERENT ETHNIC GROUPS APPROACH PALLIATIVE CARE?

Recently, more literature has been published recognizing the value of cultural competency as well as spiritual and religious awareness in patient care. A study done through the University of Miami School of Medicine surveyed 139 African American, Hispanic, and White patients to explore how these factors influence advance care directives and end-of-life decisions.[18] These patients primarily had cardiovascular and pulmonary illnesses, and a small subset carried a cancer diagnosis. Only 14% of these patients had discussions with their doctors about their treatment options while 54% desired to engage in these conversations. African American and Hispanic patients generally opted for aggressive, life-prolonging treatments despite the extent of their illness. Of all 3 groups, White patients were most likely to forgo aggressive interventions if they are diagnosed with a terminal illness.[18]

Often, cultural influences in medical care can appear to be in opposition to various ethical principles. The Patient Self-Determination Act of 1991 upheld the ethical principles of patient autonomy, informed decision making, and truth telling.[19] Patient autonomy upholds the right of an individual to make his or her own medical decisions, although this can conflict with the family structure and values of several cultures.

A study conducted in Los Angeles, California, interviewed 200 people age 65 and older who identified as European American, African American, Korean American, and Mexican American.[20] Korean American and Mexican American participants were less likely to believe that patients were told the truth about diagnosis and prognosis. It appears that older participants and those in lower socioeconomic status opposed the idea of patient autonomy more than those who were more acclimated to Western culture. Another study conducted in Boston, Massachusetts, focusing on Latino and Cambodian patients illustrated similar themes. Only 15% of these patients discussed advance care directives with their physicians in community health centers.[11] Family involvement was important for most patients: for the Latino cohort this involved their extended family, whereas for the Cambodian cohort this involved their spouse and children.

THE IMPORTANCE OF FAMILY IN DECISION MAKING

Family involvement with managing and participating in care is considered to be a basic duty. Patients who appear unengaged may have decided they do not want to decide for themselves. They also may feel they earned the right to pass decision making over to the extended family knowing they will be cared for. It can be viewed as burdensome to give honest information directly to the patient. Information can be given to family members who can then filter the information to the patient if that is what the patient desires. Interdependence is very important in several cultures and can also impact decision making. As a result, the ethical principle of beneficence is often emphasized more in non-Western cultures and the notion of telling the truth can be interpreted as "inflicting truth."[19]

In addition to defining the family unit, there are multiple points of cultural diversity that can define an individual's approach to medical care. Ongoing conversations may be required to appreciate gender roles, care of children and the elderly, marriage and relationships, view of physicians, view of suffering, and views on death and the afterlife.[21]

BARRIERS TO COMMUNICATION, ESPECIALLY AT THE END OF LIFE

Nondisclosure to the patient is more prevalent in non-Western cultures for several reasons including, but not limited to the following:

1. The view that discussion of serious illness and death is ill-mannered and barbaric
2. The concern that such discussions can lead to depression, anxiety, or other mental health concerns
3. The worry that all hope will be lost
4. The concern that speaking about illness and death will certainly cause these to become true
5. Avoidance of unnecessarily burdening elders of the community when they are ill[3]

HOW DO I BRING IT UP?

It is an incredibly daunting task to learn about all the different cultures in the world and how this can impact an individual's approach to medical care. It is important to remember that there can be regional nuances to communication and decision making so generalizations and stereotypes should be avoided. The following approach can be helpful to learn more about a new patient and how the patient goes about decision making:

1. Listen actively to appreciate how the patient understands the illness and how this is affecting the patient and the patient's family as a whole. This allows the clinician to establish a trusting relationship with the patient and the patient's family and allows them to discuss their expectations in care.
2. "Everyone is different when it comes to receiving information about their medical condition. Some people prefer to have the team speak directly to them, some would like us to speak with their families, while others prefer a combination of the two. What would you prefer?"
   - Don't be surprised if this is met with resistance. This is an opportunity to discuss Western values, such as informed consent, and that a patient cannot consent to an intervention if the patient does not know the diagnosis, disease trajectory, and prognosis.
   - In many cultures, the family, not the patient alone, comprises the decision-making locus.
3. Would you like us to speak with you regarding treatment options or is there someone else we can contact?
4. If the patient prefers to have someone else involved: Would you like us to speak with [family member] alone or while you are present[21]?

Patients have the right to change their mind, so it is imperative to readdress the preceding points to confirm the locus of decision making. In terms of speaking about the diagnosis and illness trajectory, it can be helpful to ask the following:

1. How does your family and community view sickness, treatment, pain, and death?
2. Please tell me a little about your religious beliefs. How do your religious beliefs impact your medical care?
3. Some people feel more comfortable if they are treated by someone from their own background. Are you comfortable with me taking care of you[21]?

Although some can react to the questions with a degree of suspicion, most people embrace the opportunity to share and educate others about their beliefs when they recognize the intent is good. Families may request to withhold information from the patient as a protective measure to shield the patient from the diagnosis as well as the burden of evaluating different treatment options. The patient, however, may already suspect what is going on medically and this allows the patient to discuss the topic at hand if desired. Patients may appreciate an opportunity to lead the discussions if this is not readily offered to them by their family. This also allows them the opportunity to handle unfinished business, such as completing wills, handle relationships, or return to their homeland. The family may not agree but may show better understanding if this is thoroughly explained and their loved one's wanting to take ownership of his or her decisions is continuously displayed.

UNDERSTANDING CULTURAL NORMS

Understanding various cultural norms also can make a huge difference when approaching the care of a patient. Verbal agreements are preferred and when written agreements are pursued, this can often be taken as a lack of mutual trust in a relationship. For example, if a family is in agreement with a do not resuscitate (DNR) order but seems reluctant to sign a Medical Order for Life Sustaining Treatment (MOLST), the medical team can offer to complete the form using verbal consent.

USING MEDICAL INTERPRETERS

Overcoming language barriers also can be frustrating. Most organizations have a human resources department that lists all members of the staff and the languages in which they are medically certified. Institutions also typically contract with a language interpretation company that is available with audio and/or video services. Before the conversation, interpreters should be oriented to the situation and the agenda at hand. They can provide helpful information into the cultural aspects of care. Interpreters should not be family members and are encouraged to provide word-for-word interpretation to minimize any introduction of bias into the discussion. Medical teams also should speak directly to the patient using terms such as "you" instead of "he" or "she" or "him" or "her" even when an interpreter is involved.

SUMMARY

For patients and families, addressing and exploring spiritual and cultural issues can be a source of comfort, healing, and coping during difficult times, especially at the end of life. For physicians, incorporating a patient's spirituality can potentially bring renewal, resiliency, and growth, even in difficult encounters. Sometimes as doctors we have few medical solutions for problems that cause suffering, including incurable disease, chronic pain, grief, and broken relationships. In these situations, providing this kind of comfort to patients can increase professional satisfaction and can prevent burnout.[2]

We want to leave you with this quote taken from the *Oxford Textbook on Palliative Care* that was collected by the chaplains from a nursing text:

"Spirituality is my being; my inner person. It is who I am – unique and alive. It is my body, my thinking, my feelings, my judgments, and my creativity. My spirituality motivates me to choose meaningful relationships and pursuits. Through my spirituality I give and receive love; I respond to and appreciate God, other people, a sunset, a symphony, and spring. I am driven forward, sometimes because of pain, sometimes in spite of pain. Spirituality allows me to reflect on myself. I am a person because of my spirituality – motivated and enabled to value, to worship and to communicate with the holy, the transcendent."[16]

We hope that the information offered in this article empowers you to continue giving your patients the best care possible, and to consider giving yourself the same level of compassion for your unrelenting commitment to helping those in need.

REFERENCES

1. Unruh AM, Versnel J, Kerr N. Spirituality unplugged: a review of commonalities and contentions, and resolution. Canad J Occup Ther 2002;69:15–9.
2. Saguil A, Phelps K. The spiritual assessment. Am Fam Physician 2012;86(6): 546–50.
3. Hui D, Cruz MD, Thorney S, et al. The frequency and correlates of spiritual distress among patients with advanced cancer admitted to an acute palliative care unit. Am J Hosp Palliat Care 2010;28(4):264–70.
4. Puchalski C, Ferrell B, Virani R, et al. Improving the quality of spiritual care as a dimension of palliative care: the report of the consensus conference. J Palliat Med 2009;12(10):885–904.
5. Smith-Stoner M. End-of-life preferences for atheists. J Palliat Med 2007;10(4): 923–8.
6. Mako C, Galek K, Poppito SR. Spiritual pain among patients with advanced cancer in palliative care. J Palliat Med 2006;9(5):1106–13.
7. Americans' spiritual searches turn inward. Available at: https://news.gallup.com/poll/7759/americans-spiritual-searches-turn-inward.aspx. Accessed September 15, 2018.
8. 2017 update on Americans and religion. Available at: https://news.gallup.com/poll/224642/2017-update-americans-religion.aspx. Accessed September 15, 2018.
9. Majority in U.S. still say religion can answer most problems. Available at: https://news.gallup.com/poll/211679/majority-say-religion-answer-problems.aspx. Accessed September 15, 2018.
10. Balboni TA, Vanderwerker LC, Block SD, et al. Religiousness and spiritual support among advanced cancer patients and associations with end of life treatment preferences and quality of life. J Clin Oncol 2007;25:555–60.
11. Cohen MJ, McCannon JB, Edgman-Levitan S, et al. Attitudes toward advance care directives in two diverse settings. J Palliat Med 2010;13:1427–32.
12. Richardson P. Spirituality, religion and palliative care. Ann Palliat Med 2014;3(3): 150–9.
13. Pearce MJ, Coan AD, Herndon JE 2nd, et al. Unmet spiritual care needs impact emotional and spiritual well-being in advanced cancer patients. Support Care Cancer 2012;20(10):2269–76.
14. Millspaugh CD. Assessment and response to spiritual pain: part II. J Palliat Med 2005;8(6):1110–7.
15. Puchalski CM. FICA spiritual history tool. 1996. Available at: https://smhs.gwu.edu/gwish/clinical/fica/spiritual-history-tool. Accessed October 23, 2018.
16. Harper RM III, Rudnick RE. Oxford textbook of palliative medicine. In: Hanks G, Cherny NI, Christakis NA, et al, editors. The role of the chaplain in palliative care. 4th edition. New York: Oxford University Press; 2010. p. 197–205 [Chapter 4.4].
17. "Culture." Merriam-Webster 2018. Available at: https://www.merriam-webster.com/dictionary/culture. Accessed September 10, 2018.

18. Caralis PV, Davis B, Wright K, et al. The influence of ethnicity and race on attitudes toward advance directives, life-prolonging treatments, and euthanasia. J Clin Ethics 1993;4(2):155–65.
19. Ersek M, Kagawa-Singer M, Barnes D, et al. Multicultural considerations in the use of advance directives. Oncol Nurs Forum 1998;25(10):1683–90.
20. Blackhall LJ, Murphy ST, Frank G, et al. Ethnicity and attitudes toward patient autonomy. JAMA 1995;274(10):820–5.
21. Searight HR, Gafford J. Cultural diversity at the end of life: issues and guidelines for family physicians. Am Fam Physician 2005;71(3):515–22.

Palliative Care Approach to Chronic Diseases

End Stages of Heart Failure, Chronic Obstructive Pulmonary Disease, Liver Failure, and Renal Failure

Kathleen Mechler, MD*, John Liantonio, MD

KEYWORDS

- Heart failure • COPD • ESRD • ESLD • Advance care planning
- Advanced therapies • Palliative care • Hospice care

KEY POINTS

- Palliative and hospice services are underutilized by end-stage noncancer patients.
- Patients with chronic end-stage disease have unique symptom management needs, and their management is a necessary skill for primary care physicians.
- Uncertainty makes advance care planning difficult, but prognostic tools are available. Discussions should focus on defining and preserving a minimum quality of life.
- Early hospice referral could benefit patients with symptomatic chronic end-stage conditions.

INTRODUCTION

Classically, hospice and palliative services have been most available to and disproportionately used by patients with cancer. No data exist on community outpatient palliative care availability; however, anecdotally these services are sparse, leaving the unmet palliative and end-of-life needs of end-stage chronically ill patients in the clinics of the primary care providers. These end-stage noncancer patients have their own unique management and prognostic challenges discussed in this article.

Disclosures: The authors have nothing to disclose.
Department of Family and Community Medicine, Division of Geriatric Medicine and Palliative Care, Thomas Jefferson University Hospital, 1015 Walnut Street Suite 401, Philadelphia, PA 19107, USA
* Corresponding author.
E-mail address: kathleen.mechler@jefferson.edu

Prim Care Clin Office Pract 46 (2019) 415–432
https://doi.org/10.1016/j.pop.2019.05.008
0095-4543/19/© 2019 Elsevier Inc. All rights reserved.

END-STAGE HEART FAILURE

Heart failure (HF) is a syndrome of reduced cardiac output resulting in fluid overload, edema, breathlessness, and fatigue.[1,2] HF is caused by structural or functional defects, commonly ischemic heart disease, toxins, infectious endocarditis, valve disease, systemic or pulmonary hypertension, arrhythmias, or chronic volume overload as seen in renal failure.[1] Often the cause is multifactorial or idiopathic. More than 6.5 million American adults are living with HF, a number expected to increase to greater than 8 million by 2030.[3] Heart diseases are the leading cause of death in this country, and a significant system cost is estimated conservatively at $32.9 billion but up to $115.4 billion when including all costs for patients with HF as a comorbidity. Survival has improved over decades but mortality remains high.[4,5]

HF is diagnosed using the Framingham Diagnostic Criteria with laboratory testing and echocardiography and can be characterized as either HF with preserved ejection fraction (EF) of 40% or more (HFpEF) or with reduced ejection fraction less than 40% (HFrEF). HF patients' functional status is classified American College of Cardiology Foundation/American Heart Association (ACCF/AHA) stages A to D (no symptoms to refractory) or New York Heart Association (NYHA) class I to IV (no activity limits to HF symptoms at rest).[1] The illness is progressive in symptoms and functional limitations with an unpredictable time course with or without changes in EF. End-stage HF includes patients of ACCF/AHA stage D or NYHA class IV with symptoms at rest.

Symptom Management

HF patients are often initially managed in the primary care office, and the goal of treatment is to reduce symptoms and mortality. Initial treatment should always include management of comorbidities and lifestyle. Pharmacologic therapy for HFrEF should include an angiotensin-converting enzyme inhibitor and β-blocker with consideration for additional medications, such as mineralocorticoid receptor antagonist, diuretics, angiotensin receptor blockers, hydralazine with isosorbide, and newer medications, such as angiotensin receptor neprilysin inhibitors and I_f-channel inhibitors. HFpEF has less research and guidelines, but diuretics do improve symptoms with some evidence supporting mineralocorticoid receptor antagonist (MRAs) and β-blockers.[2,6] The following are treatment recommendations for symptoms refractory to standard treatments.

Dyspnea is the most common complaint of HF patients and is present in 86% of patients in the last year of life.[7] When diuresis is optimized or limited by hypotension and side effects, low-dose opioids, such as oral morphine 2.5 to 5 mg every 4 to 6 hours, can decrease breathlessness and have little risk aside from constipation.[5,8,9] Benzodiazepines have a similar but nonsignificant effect but with higher risk of mortality so are second-line therapy.[10] Oxygen is only beneficial in reducing dyspnea in the setting of hypoxemia.[5]

Lower-extremity edema is present in most patients at end of life, and if refractory to diuresis, there are few effective treatments. Treat with skin care and pain management as needed. Pain is another common symptom in HF at end of life. Nonsteroidal anti-inflammatory medications can be contraindicated with common comorbidities so at end of life low-dose opioids are reasonable and safe.[5] Avoid the use of methadone because of its QTc prolonging effect.

Fatigue is a distressing symptom that can be found in 39% of newly diagnosed patients as well as 57% of end-stage HF patients.[7,11] Fatigue is associated with depression, and prevalence of both increases with increased symptom burden.[11,12] Unfortunately, evidence on how to treat depression in HF is limited, so selective serotonin reuptake inhibitors (SSRIs) are still considered first-line therapy along with cognitive behavior therapy (CBT). Tricyclic antidepressants (TCAs) are not recommended because of QTc prolongation and anticholinergic side effects.[5,13,14]

Prognostication

Prognostication in HF is difficult with unpredictable exacerbations and rates of decline. Multiple tools are available to assist in prediction of hospitalization or all-cause mortality for HF patients. The variables impacting prognosis include age, creatinine, blood pressure, sodium level, EF, sex, cardiac biomarkers, NYHA class, diabetes, and weight. No 1 tool is superior, so use by applicability.[2,15–18] Models are based on population data, and clinical experience should be used to personalize this prediction (**Table 1**).

Advanced Therapies

An implantable cardioverter-defibrillator (ICD) is recommended for the primary and secondary prevention of death from arrhythmias in advanced HF with EF less than 30%. ICDs do not improve symptoms, but they do prolong life and should be considered if prognosis is more than 1 year.[2]

Continuous inotrope infusions of milrinone or dobutamine for palliation are controversial. Use has either neutral or negative impact on mortality with median survival of 9 months and mixed evidence of symptom improvement.[19–23] Inotrope infusion remains recommended because of case-based evidence of symptom improvement and is reserved for cardiogenic hypotension with a goal of bridging to mechanical support or home for palliation.[24] With a peripherally inserted central catheter, an infusion company for medication and equipment, and adequate emergency help at home, a

Table 1 Prognostic indices for heart failure		
What Score Predicts	**Index**	**Variables Included**
In-hospital mortality	GWTG-HF	Blood pressure, BUN, sodium, age, pulse, COPD history, black race
1–5 y mortality or risk of hospitalization	BCN Bio-HF	Age, sex, NYHA class, sodium, eGFR, hemoglobin, EF, HF duration, diabetes, number of HF hospitalizations in last year, diuretic amount, statin, β-blocker, ACEI/ARB. ARNi, CRT, ICD, cardiac biomarkers (troponin, ST2, NT-proBNP)
	3C-HF	NYHA class, atrial fibrillation, severe valve disease, EF, comorbidities (anemia, complicated diabetes, hypertension, creatinine), age, BB, ACEI ARB
	Seattle Heart Failure Model	Age, sex, NYHA class, weight, EF, systolic blood pressure, ischemic heart disease, ACEI, BB, ARB, statin, allopurinol, aldosterone blocker, diuretics dose, hemoglobin lymphocyte %, uric acid, total cholesterol, sodium, ECG abnormalities, pressors or inotropes use, cardiac devices (CRT, ICD, IABP, LVAD)

Abbreviations: ACEI, angiotensin-converting enzyme inhibitor; ARB, angiotensin II receptor blocker; ARNi, angiotensin receptor-neprilysin inhibitor; BB, β-blocker; BCN Bio-HF, Barcelona bio-heart failure; BUN, blood urea nitrogen; 3C-HF, cardiac and comorbid conditions–heart failure; ECG, electrocardiogram; eGFR, estimated glomerular filtration rate; GWTG-HF, get with the guidelines–heart failure; HF, heart failure; IABP, intra-aortic balloon pump; LBBB, left bundle branch block; LVAD, left ventricular assist device; NT-proBNP, N-terminal pro B-type naturetic peptide.
Data from Refs.[2,15–18]

patient can be discharged home with inotropes. Select hospices will support this treatment. If inadequate social support or follow-up, use should be limited to a trial in-hospital.

Mechanical support is offered when inotropic support is insufficient. Cardiac resynchronization therapy (CRT) with a biventricular pacemaker can improve pumping, allowing improved functional class, quality of life, and for select patients, improved mortality.[24,25] Select medical centers offer left ventricular assist devices (LVADs) to provide the power for cardiac output implanted either as a bridge to cardiac transplantation or as a destination therapy (DT). LVADs can improve survival and quality of life with DT survival exceeding 50% at 3 years, but disappointingly, a high percentage of patients encounter complications causing decreased quality and survival.[3] Informed consent for LVAD should include these risks, discussion of minimal quality of life desired, and the right to deactivate the pump.[26,27]

Cardiac transplant is offered to refractory patients without significant comorbidity and offers real survival benefit. Median survival has improved now to 10.7 years even as the proportion of patients transplanted over the age of 60 has increased. Studies show long-term posttransplant improvement in quality of life and function, but that younger patients find limitations bothersome at 1 year and require treatment of symptoms, especially depression.[28]

Advance Care Planning and End-of-Life Care

Guidelines advocate strongly for early and repeated discussions of prognosis and goals of care. Discussion of prognosis includes if disease follows its natural course and the risk of sudden events at all phases of illness. Care planning should include naming a health care proxy, a plan for sudden events, and a plan to define and preserve a minimum quality of life. When patients are at an intolerable quality of life on advanced treatments or are at end of life, the following comfort-focused care changes can prevent suffering. Deactivation of ICD is recommended to avoid nonbeneficial shocks at end of life, done by device representatives or by placing a strong magnet over the unit. Deactivation of CRT is not necessary unless requested because of patient suffering. Withdrawal of inotropes or LVAD should be done in a hospital or hospice prepared to use opioids for dyspnea. Time to death after cessation of inotropes is variable, although likely hours to days, and likely minutes after LVAD deactivation.[5]

END-STAGE CHRONIC OBSTRUCTIVE PULMONARY DISEASE

Chronic obstructive pulmonary disease (COPD) encompasses the illnesses emphysema and chronic bronchitis, both progressive respiratory conditions characterized by incompletely reversible airflow obstructions from inflammation and parenchymal destruction.[29] The most common cause by far is smoking; other causes include other toxic exposures, severe recurrent infections, and inherited conditions, such as alpha-1 antitrypsin deficiency (A1AD).[29,30] COPD affects 12 to 15 million American adults with another likely 12 million undiagnosed.[31–33] Trends in prevalence show disproportionate burden of disease in women and rural areas.[33,34] Chronic lower respiratory illnesses are the fourth most common cause of death in the United States, expected to be third by 2020.[32,35] The total cost burden of COPD nears $36 billion with expected increase to $49 billion by 2020.[36]

Diagnosis is suspected when a patient with a smoking history complains of progressive dyspnea or chronic cough and is confirmed with spirometry revealing persistent post–inhaler airflow limitation with forced expiratory volume in 1 second (FEV_1)/forced vital capacity value less than 0.70 of predicted value.[30] Illness severity is classified by the Global Initiative for Chronic Obstructive Lung Disease (GOLD) Score and Redefined ABCD Assessment Tool. The FEV_1 decrease determines the GOLD score from mild (1; $\geq$80%) to severe (4; <30%), and history of exacerbations and hospitalizations with a dyspnea assessment is used in a grid to give a grouping A (minimal symptoms) to D (multiple exacerbations with high dyspnea burden).[30] Patients classified as GOLD 4 and group D are considered end stage.

Symptom Management

Many COPD treatments can improve symptoms, improve quality of life, and increase longevity.[31] In early and all stages of COPD, management should include smoking cessation, vaccines, short-acting bronchodilators with or without long-acting bronchodilators to prevent or reduce symptoms, and inhaled corticosteroids to reduce exacerbations.[30] Intermittent oral steroids for 5 days and antibiotic treatments are indicated in exacerbations of disease.[37] The progression of COPD is variable, and standard behavioral and medical interventions can control symptoms for years, but as illness severity increases, it may be necessary to refer to specialty pulmonary care to consider advanced medical and interventional therapies. Medications include phosphodiesterase-4 inhibitors and A1AD augmentation therapy. Use of chronic oral steroids or antibiotics is reserved for patients with frequent exacerbations given the risk of harm and resistance.[30,38] The following are treatment recommendations for symptoms refractory to medical management.

Dyspnea is the most common complaint in advanced COPD present in almost all patients in the last year of life. It causes 45% of patients to be homebound and 75% to require a caregiver, and this dyspnea can be more severe and for a more prolonged time than in end-stage lung cancer.[39–41] Dyspnea is impacted by multiple factors producing physiologic and behavioral responses, and treatment at end of life is imperative for quality of life.[42] Opioids reduce discomfort of air hunger and are the treatment of choice in severe disease. Improvement can be seen with as little as 2.5 to 5 mg oral morphine with evidence that safe titration up to 30 mg morphine daily can provide 35% improvement from baseline breathlessness.[10,43] Despite the strong recommendation, studies show only 2% of stable outpatient patients with COPD and 25% of palliative patients with COPD are prescribed opioids compared with half of patients with lung cancer.[44,45] This underuse could lead to undue suffering at end of life. Side effects are usually minimal at low doses. Benzodiazepines are reserved for second-line treatment.[10,46] Inhaled furosemide is being studied for treatment of breathlessness, but at this time there is not enough evidence to support use.[42] Mucolytics, such as N-acetylcysteine, expectorants, such as guaifenesin, or antitussives, such as benzonatate, have poor efficacy data; however, they are well tolerated, and case studies report improvement in quality of life.[35,47,48] A small study did find a significant improvement in breathlessness with the use of a simple handheld fan directed at the face, but oxygen use without hypoxia is not helpful.[43,49] Oxygen is indicated in the treatment of advanced COPD with severe resting hypoxemia and use for more than 15 hours daily increases survival.[31,42,50,51]

Fatigue is the second most prevalent symptom in early and late disease, and extreme fatigue is comparable to amyotrophic lateral sclerosis.[39,52] The most effect intervention is pulmonary rehabilitation with at least 4 weeks of exercise training plus education or psychological support. Additional benefits include improved dyspnea, emotional function, patients' sense of control over their breathing, and improved health-related quality of life.[30,53,54] Disappointingly, this effective intervention is only available to approximately 2% of the COPD population.[55]

Mood symptoms are another common complaint and are more prevalent than in the general population.[39,53,56] Undertreatment endangers patients because uncontrolled depression is associated with medication noncompliance, more frequent exacerbations and hospitalizations, and greater mortality.[35] However, despite the severity of symptoms, patients exhibited low desire for death and an overall absence of suicidal ideation, likely due to the slow progression of illness allowing for adaptation to the disability and decreasing quality of life.[52] Patients should be screened for depression at each visit in order to consider treatment. Strongest nonpharmacologic efficacy data exist for pulmonary rehabilitation in improving depression as well as for CBT reducing anxiety.[52,53] Insignificant evidence exists to recommend other than standard treatment, such as SSRI or TCAs (caution in elderly) for depression and buspar for anxiety. Consider benzodiazepines only with palliative intent due to increased risk of death.[52,53,57,58]

Pain is another symptom more prevalent in the patients with COPD than in the general population.[39,59,60] Comorbidities and dyspnea are risk factors, and comorbidities are likely to limit nonopioid medications. Pain in early disease in the absence of dyspnea should be treated conservatively; however, opioids should be considered in advanced disease with severe dyspnea.

Prognostication

COPD includes variably progressive respiratory illnesses for which it is difficult to prognosticate. Only dementia is shown to have a more unpredictable clinical course.[53] FEV_1 alone is inadequate for prognostication, so several survival indexes were developed to give meaningful prognostic information using body mass index (BMI), FEV_1, dyspnea scales, exercise capacity, exacerbations, and comorbidities. All tools are useful in helping patients and families make decisions about advanced treatment options but should be combined with clinician experience[61,62] (**Table 2**).

Advanced Therapies

Patients with severe emphysema can have improved outcomes with lung volume reduction surgery (LVRS) to remove space-occupying damaged lung that shunts air from healthy lung. Surgery is most beneficial for patients with severe upper lobe emphysema and poor functional capacity offering improved exercise capacity,

Table 2		
Prognostic indices for chronic obstructive pulmonary disease		
Index	**Use**	**Variables**
BODE	Most validated index	BMI, airflow obstruction, dyspnea by MMRC, exercise capacity
	Predicts 1- to 5-y mortality in stable outpatients	
	Highest scores indicate 1-y 5% and 5-y 80% mortality	
CODEX	Predicts 3- and 12-mo mortality; higher scores 6–9 indicate 5%–10% and 20%–30% mortality, respectively, whereas a score of 10 indicates 22% and 55% mortalities	Comorbidities, airway obstruction, dyspnea by MMRC, number of exacerbations per year

Abbreviations: BODEX, body mass index (BMI), airflow obstruction, Dyspnea measured by Medical Research Council (MMRC) scale, and Exercise capacity by distance walked in 6 minutes; CODEX, Comorbidity by Charleston index, airway Obstruction, Dyspnea by MMRC, and number of EXacerbations.

Data from Celli BR, Cote CG, Marin JM, et al. The body-mass index, airflow obstruction, dyspnea, and exercise capacity index in chronic obstructive pulmonary disease. N Engl J Med 2004;350(10):1005–12; and Almagro P, Soriano JB, Cabrera FJ, et al. Short- and medium-term prognosis in patients hospitalized for COPD exacerbation: the CODEX index. Chest 2014;145(5):972–80.

quality of life, and survival. For all other patients not meeting these criteria, the outcomes are worse than medical management, so surgery is not recommended.[30,63,64] An endobronchial valve procedure has similar outcomes with a low complication rate; however, treatment failure is also higher, so more research is required.[65,66] LVRS is not recommended as a bridge to transplant as subsequent outcomes are worse.[67]

Noninvasive positive pressure ventilation (NPPV) is a form of mechanical support using oxygen delivered with positive pressure that can be applied by nasal device or face mask; examples include CPAP and BiPAP. Use in acute COPD exacerbations reduces mortality by 46% and need for intubation by 65% and decreases hospital length of stay.[68] There is no mortality benefit to routine home use in stable COPD; it is only recommended and covered by insurance in patients with COPD with certain criteria.[35] Treatment intolerance limits NPPV use but is standard of care in hospital-based treatment of severe exacerbations and should be offered to all patients regardless of their desire for invasive mechanical ventilation (MV). MV is offered to patients requiring more support for hypoxia or hypercapnia. Use can be short in patients with COPD with median of 3 days use, and intensive care unit (ICU) mortality of 9% to 16% is lower for vented patients with COPD than if on MV for other reasons.[69,70] Survival statistics can be encouraging for patients and families; however, untold in these numbers is the significant post-ICU morbidity, including debility and risk for readmission.

At a few advanced centers, extracorporeal support is available for temporary use as a bridge to lung transplantation. The process is similar to dialysis with blood filtered through an external circuit and includes the technologies of extracorporeal membrane oxygenation and extracorporeal carbon dioxide removal. These extracorporeal treatments are used with the intention of avoiding MV and ventilator-induced lung injury, and in some cases, the patient can be ambulatory to avoid ICU debility. Small studies show high mortality but earlier extubation and mobilization with good results after transplantation and complication rates similar to any central venous catheter.[71,72]

Lung transplant is an option for select advanced patients with COPD who have progressive disease despite optimal treatments. Bilateral lung transplants offer better outcomes than single lung, and a transplant can improve health status, quality of life, and functional capacity.[30,67] Data regarding survival are disappointing, with high short-term mortality and no statistical evidence of survival benefit for most patients with COPD with the exception of A1AD or BMI, airflow obstruction, dyspnea, exercise capacity (BODE≥7).[73,74] Experts believe transplant is still beneficial in COPD patients due to improved quality of life regardless of neutral mortality impact; however, patients and families must weigh this benefit against the very real risk of high short-term mortality. Recent survival data show median survival for patients with COPD after transplant is 5.7 years, increasing to 7.9 years for recipients who survive the first year.[75]

Advance Care Planning and End-of-Life Care

Many patients will not be eligible for, have access to, or choose not to use the treatments above with the exception of MV. Decisions about treatments should start in the outpatient setting with a discussion of likely prognosis and outcomes.[30] Barriers include clinician difficulty in prognosticating as well as a patient prognostic or disease-related disbelief given previous personal recovery or observing other variable illness courses.[53,56,76] As a consequence compared with patients with cancer, patients with COPD are less likely to have documented goals of care conversations, have longer hospital and ICU stays, and are more likely to have CPR and no DNR at end of life.[40] A survey of advanced patients with COPD identified milestones that may trigger discussions: loss of hobbies, a change in the home to accommodate illness, increased episodes of acute care, initiation of home oxygen, a need for assistance with self-care, and panic attacks.[77] Start by recommending a health care proxy; patients should share with their proxy their desire for minimal quality of life and their decisions regarding life support if that quality of life cannot realistically be achieved. If the most likely outcome of an intervention is not desired, then the proxy has the right to make decisions to withdraw life support, typically the ventilator. The patient with COPD undergoing MV withdrawal is at risk for severe dyspnea and should be treated in a hospital or hospice setting with access to parenteral opioids and medications to treat secretions; prognosis will be variable, but likely hours to days.

END-STAGE RENAL DISEASE

Progression of patients to end-stage renal disease (ESRD) from chronic kidney disease (CKD) is difficult to predict. Many patients with the disease will remain in CKD I–V, whereas some may progress to ESRD. CKD is considered to be present in patients with glomerular filtration rate (GFR) less than 60 mL/min, whereas ESRD can be recognized in patients with GFR less than 15 mL/min. Quite often, patients with CKD are at higher risk of mortality associated with cardiovascular disease because the presence of CKD alone should be considered a coronary risk equivalent.[78]

ESRD is seen in more than 650,000 patients per year in the United States and 2 million patients worldwide. This number is increasing 5% annually in the United States. The cost associated with treating ESRD is staggering, with hemodialysis costing $89,000 per patient annually, amounting to $42 billion in the United States. Although only 1% of the Medicare population has ESRD, it makes up about 7% of the annual budget.[79]

Symptom Management

Patients suffering with ESRD often display symptoms of the sensations of fluid overload as well as uremia. Although the focus in CKD is identification of reversible causes of worsening kidney disease, the focus in ESRD is symptomatic management.

Fluid overload is managed with reduction in sodium intake as well as use of loop diuretics, furosemide and bumetanide. Unfortunately, the effect of diuretics is often limited in the patient with ESRD because many of those patients are oliguric or anuric in end stage. Fluid restriction can be attempted but is often poorly tolerated due to impact on quality of life.

In uremic patients, typical symptoms include delirium, fatigue, nausea, vomiting, anorexia, and malnutrition. Management in this setting often involves management of the individual symptoms. For further discussion on management of these individual symptoms, see the general article on symptom management.

Pruritus may pose another problem. Providers should attempt topical treatment first with moisturizers, which can often be very effective. Doxepin can be helpful as well, but its use is often limited due to risk of delirium. Other medications shown effective are mirtazapine 15 to 30 mg daily and gabapentin 300 mg.[80]

Prognostication

Prognostication in patients with ESRD is typically very challenging. Although some patients progress from CKD to ESRD, not all will. Of those patients with ESRD, it is difficult to predict onset of death from diagnosis of ESRD. Typically, patients undergoing renal replacement therapy have longer life expectancy than those opting for conservative therapy. Patients in the conservative cohort typically have a life expectancy of 6 to 24 months, with the median survival being 6 months.[81]

Advanced Therapies

Although there are many mechanisms to manage symptoms associated with ESRD, definitive therapy typically involves the initiation of hemodialysis. Patients undergoing hemodialysis are required to receive therapy multiple times a week, typically at a dialysis center. Indications to initiate dialysis include pericarditis, progressive encephalopathy, resistant hypertension, and persistent metabolic disturbances. To prevent life-threatening complications related to ESRD, many nephrologists will initiate dialysis when GFR is less than 10 mL/min.[82]

Advance Care Planning and End-of-Life Care

Conservative management of ESRD is often indicated in patients who will not see the full benefit of dialysis either because of overwhelming comorbidities or limited life expectancy. The Renal Physicians Association recommends conservative management for patients older than 75 years with impaired functional status, severe malnutrition, multiple comorbidities, or those whose physicians answer no to the surprise question: "would you be surprised if this patient died within 1 year?"[83] It is also important to match patients' goals to the treatment plan. The authors recommend an extensive goals-of-care discussion involving both patients and their family/caregivers. A realistic picture of what is involved with dialysis, including transportation, many hours spent at dialysis centers, and the risks involved with dialysis, must be discussed in detail when discussing desire for dialysis.

Conservative therapy, or intent to defer dialysis, is a treatment modality that as described above should be considered in patients with significant disease burden, comorbidities, or simply those patients who do not wish to undertake dialysis. Elderly patients are of particular concern here. These patients are at significant risk of delayed recovery following dialysis sessions, and many patients describe more than 6 hours to recover.[84] Depression is also common among this group, with older dialysis patients having a 62% increased risk of developing depression.[85] There is also 3 times the mortality risk within 1 year of initiation of dialysis among frail elderly patients.[86] Management of elderly dialysis patients must include a specific discussion of the significant morbidity and mortality.

Patients opting for cessation of dialysis after being on dialysis for months typically are faced with a life expectancy of 7 to 14 days. The authors recommend sharing this prognosis as in all disease states in terms of hours to days or days to weeks rather than giving specific numbers because families often struggle with the specifics of this information. Death by cessation of hemodialysis is typically well tolerated and can be managed medically. Providers should be diligent to the presence of pulmonary edema and associated dyspnea and be treated with opioids. Many patients will also display signs and symptoms of delirium. Ultimately, patients dying of ESRD will become comatose and should be managed accordingly. Care for the comatose patient can be accomplished at home, or often in an inpatient hospice setting, because disease burden can be high for families or caregivers.

END-STAGE LIVER DISEASE

End-stage liver disease (ESLD) is typically seen in patients with liver failure or decompensated cirrhosis. Patients with decompensated cirrhosis display signs and symptoms of liver failure, including variceal bleeds, ascites, spontaneous bacterial peritonitis (SBP), and hepatorenal syndrome (HRS).[87] ESLD is considered the 12th leading cause of death in the United States, accounting for 40,326 deaths in 2015.[88] Cirrhosis can also have several causes, including hepatitis B (15%), hepatitis C (47%), and alcohol use (18%).[89]

As in many chronic conditions, cost is a major factor because illnesses such as ESLD can cause a huge burden to health care systems. For patients with no cirrhosis, annual costs can be estimated to be $17,277, increasing to $22,752 with compensated cirrhosis, and $59,995 annually for ESLD.[90] This illness also can pose a severe strain to hospital systems in that patients have a high likelihood for multiple hospitalizations, accounting for approximately 150,000 hospitalizations annually. Hospitalizations and cost are considered to be even higher in patients who are transplanted. There are about 6000 patients receiving transplant annually with costs being in the hundreds of thousands of dollars for care before, during, and after transplantation.[91]

Symptom Management

Symptoms associated with ESLD are attributed to toxin buildup causing an altered mental status. There are 2 approaches to addressing acute encephalopathy. First, search for reversible causes, including infection, hypovolemia, renal failure, HF, medication side effects, and electrolyte disturbances.[92] Second, focus should be on reduction of blood ammonia, which may be accounting for changes in mental status. Initiation of lactulose at 20 to 30 g given 2 to 4 times daily should be the first step. Treatment is measured as effective based on frequency of bowel movements. Disaccharide drugs like rifaximin should be used in conjunction with lactulose for prevention of encephalopathy at doses of 400 mg 2 to 3 times daily.[93]

For patients who are unable to have their encephalopathy delirium managed with the above approaches, more aggressive symptom management is necessary. Often this requires one-on-one staffing if hospitalized or in a long-term care facility. However, the use of antipsychotic, benzodiazepine, or barbiturate medications should be considered for the safety of both patient and staff. Discussion with the patient's medical decision maker is often necessary before initiating these medications because they can be very sedating for patients.

Another common challenge in patients with ESLD is ascites. Although in patients with cardiac or renal deficiencies diuretics are often the mainstay of therapy, these drugs are often ineffective because patients are intravascularly depleted because of low concentrations of albumin in the intravascular space. Similarly, many patients with ESLD suffer with comorbid renal failure whereby diuretics are less effective. However, if using a diuretic is necessary due to limited options, spironolactone is the preferred drug of choice because it is not protein bound like furosemide.[94] Dietary restriction of sodium to less than 2000 mg daily plus fluid restriction may also be effective, but evidence is poor.[95]

Pruritus from hyperbilirubinemia is often a common complaint. Management should be done similarly to above discussion with the addition of cholestyramine.[96]

Prognostication

To best understand severity and life expectancy in patients with ESLD, it is necessary to know the Model for End-Stage Liver Disease (MELD) score. The score uses serum bilirubin, serum creatinine, and international normalized ratio (INR) to predict the chance of 3-month mortality. Some models include serum sodium as a factor. As MELD score increases, 3-month survival decreases (**Table 3**). This tool is also used to help determine organ allocation and where patients may fall on the transplant list. Patients with higher MELD scores are considered to be sicker and therefore may receive preference for organ transplant. Interestingly, time on transplant list is used to break ties in patients with the same MELD score and blood type.[97]

What makes prognostication a further dilemma is that there are potentially curable treatments available for many of the causes of liver disease. With the introduction of

Table 3	
Model for end-stage liver disease score and associated mortality	
MELD Score	**90-day Mortality (90%)**
$\geq$40	71.3
30–39	52.6
20–29	19.6
10–19	6
$\leq$9	1.9

MELD Formula = 3.78 × ln[serum bilirubin (mg/dL)] + 11.2 × ln[INR] + 9.57 × ln[serum creatine (mg/mL)] + 6.43.
  Data from Biggins SW, Bambha K. MELD-based liver allocation: who is underserved? Semin Liver Dis 2006;26(3):211–20.

interferon and direct-acting antiviral agents, hepatitis C virus can be eradicated from patients, resulting in some reversal of cirrhosis symptoms.[98] In addition, transplant can cure cirrhosis through replacement with a healthy liver. However, as noted above, only a limited number of patients ever reach transplant. The authors recommend consultation with hepatology teams in management and transplant decision making for this complicated population.

Advanced Therapies

When dietary and diuretic management are ineffective, patients are considered to have diuretic-resistant ascites, and this is often managed with paracentesis or a trans-jugular intrahepatic portosystemic shunt (TIPS). The TIPS procedure has risks of infection, bleeding, and clotting of shunt and is reserved for patients with a MELD score of less than 18 who cannot tolerate large-volume paracentesis.[99] An indwelling tunneled peritoneal catheter is an option for easier fluid withdrawal in patients requiring more frequent paracentesis; however, this is reserved for patients who are no longer transplant eligible and have a limited life expectancy of weeks to months. Catheters are placed by Interventional Radiology or Hepatology before discharge from a hospital setting, and it allows patients to avoid repeat procedures and drain at home. It is typically reserved for hospice patients whereby the benefits in aiding discomfort related to ascites outweighs associated increased risk of infection.[100]

Use of a molecular adsorbent recirculation system for patients with advanced decompensated liver disease is on the increase in many inpatient settings, serving as a type of liver dialysis. Although this treatment can potentially show some reversal in laboratory abnormalities commonly seen in this population, evidence supporting widespread use is conflicting. Current use is limited to patients who are critically ill requiring hospitalization.[101,102]

HOSPICE FOR CHRONIC CONDITIONS

Uncertainty over when to refer patients to hospice is often cited as one of the barriers to earlier hospice referral.[103] The authors recommend partnering with local hospice medical directors or palliative care teams where available to assist in a consultative role to identify patients who may benefit from early hospice referral. Published hospice criteria for end-stage conditions are only a guideline for when to consider referral; however, not meeting these criteria is not a contraindication to qualification or referral (**Table 4**). Earlier referral is recommended for patients with multiple comorbidities, heavy symptom burden, and comfort-focused goals.

Table 4
Hospice criteria

Disease	Hospice Criteria
COPD	• Disabling dyspnea at rest, little or no response to bronchodilators, decreased functional capacity & • Progression of disease as evidenced by increasing health care utilization & • Hypoxemia at rest with oxygen saturation <88%
CHF	• NYHA class IV and significant symptoms at rest • EF of <20% • Patient is on optimal treatment • Patient has angina at rest, no longer a candidate for other treatments
ESRD	• Patient is not seeking or is not a candidate for hemodialysis • Creatinine clearance <15 mL/min • Serum creatinine >6 mg/dL
ESLD	• PT >5 s or INR >1.5 • Albumin <2.5 g/dL • Refractory ascites, h/o SBP, HRS, refractory hepatic encephalopathy, recurrent variceal bleed

Abbreviations: CHF, congestive heart failure; PT, prothrombin time.

Data from Gentle Shepherd Hospice. Hospice eligibility criteria. Available at: https://gentleshepherdhospice.com/wp-content/uploads/2018/07/Hospice_elegibility_card__Ross_and_Sanchez_Reilly_2008.pdf.

REFERENCES

1. Yancy CW, Jessup M, Bozkurt B, et al. 2013 ACCF/AHA guideline for the management of heart failure: executive summary: a report of the American College of Cardiology Foundation/American Heart Association Task Force on practice guidelines. Circulation 2013;128(16):1810–52.

2. Ponikowski P, Voors AA, Anker SD, et al. 2016 ESC guidelines for the diagnosis and treatment of acute and chronic heart failure. The Task Force for the diagnosis and treatment of acute and chronic heart failure of the European Society of Cardiology (ESC) developed with the special contribution of the Heart Failure Association (HFA) of the ESC. Eur Heart J 2016;37(27):2129–200.

3. Benjamin EJ, Virani SS, Callaway CW, et al. Heart disease and stroke statistics—2018 update: a report from the American Heart Association. Circulation 2018. Available at: http://www.ahajournals.org/doi/abs/10.1161/CIR.0000000000000558. Accessed October 7, 2018.

4. Voigt J, Sasha John M, Taylor A, et al. A reevaluation of the costs of heart failure and its implications for allocation of health resources in the United States. Clin Cardiol 2014;37(5):312–21.

5. LeMond L, Allen LA. Palliative care and hospice in advanced heart failure. Prog Cardiovasc Dis 2011;54(2):168–78.

6. Martin N, Manoharan K, Thomas J, et al. Beta-blockers and inhibitors of the renin-angiotensin aldosterone system for chronic heart failure with preserved ejection fraction. Cochrane Database Syst Rev 2018;(6):CD012721.

7. Voon V, Chew S, Craig C, et al. Can we do better in improving end of life care and symptom control in end-stage heart failure? Heart 2017;103(Suppl 6):A4.

8. Johnson MJ, McDonagh TA, Harkness A, et al. Morphine for the relief of breathlessness in patients with chronic heart failure—a pilot study. Eur J Heart Fail 2002;4(6):753–6.

9. Goodlin SJ. Palliative care in congestive heart failure. J Am Coll Cardiol 2009; 54(5):386–96.

10. Ekström MP, Bornefalk-Hermansson A, Abernethy AP, et al. Safety of benzodiazepines and opioids in very severe respiratory disease: national prospective study. BMJ 2014;348.

11. Williams BA. The clinical epidemiology of fatigue in newly diagnosed heart failure. BMC Cardiovasc Disord 2017;17(1):122.

12. Rutledge T, Reis VA, Linke SE, et al. Depression in heart failure a meta-analytic review of prevalence, intervention effects, and associations with clinical outcomes. J Am Coll Cardiol 2006;48(8):1527–37.

13. O'Connor CM, Jiang W, Kuchibhatla M, et al. Safety and efficacy of sertraline for depression in patients with heart failure: results of the SADHART-CHF (Sertraline Against Depression and Heart Disease in Chronic Heart Failure) trial. J Am Coll Cardiol 2010;56(9):692–9.

14. Joynt KE, O'Connor CM. Lessons from SADHART, ENRICHD, and other trials. Psychosom Med 2005;67(Suppl 1):S63–6.

15. Rahimi K, Bennett D, Conrad N, et al. Risk prediction in patients with heart failure: a systematic review and analysis. JACC Heart Fail 2014;2(5):440–6.

16. Levy WC, Mozaffarian D, Linker DT, et al. The Seattle Heart Failure Model: prediction of survival in heart failure. Circulation 2006;113(11):1424–33.

17. Senni M, Parrella P, De Maria R, et al. Predicting heart failure outcome from cardiac and comorbid conditions: the 3C-HF score. Int J Cardiol 2013;163(2): 206–11.

18. Peterson PN, Rumsfeld JS, Liang L, et al. A validated risk score for in-hospital mortality in patients with heart failure from the American Heart Association Get With the Guidelines Program. Circ Cardiovasc Qual Outcomes 2010;3(1): 25–32.

19. Guglin M, Kaufman M. Inotropes do not increase mortality in advanced heart failure. Int J Gen Med 2014;7:237–51.

20. Hashim T, Sanam K, Revilla-Martinez M, et al. Clinical characteristics and outcomes of intravenous inotropic therapy in advanced heart failure. Circ Heart Fail 2015;8(5):880–6.

21. Mortara A, Oliva F, Metra M, et al. Treatment with inotropes and related prognosis in acute heart failure: contemporary data from the Italian Network on Heart Failure (IN-HF) Outcome registry. J Heart Lung Transplant 2014;33(10):1056–65.

22. Cardoso JN, Grossi A, Del Carlo CH, et al. Mortality rates are going down in clinical use of inotropics. Temporal trends for prognosis in acute decompensated heart failure (1992/1999–2005/2006). Int J Cardiol 2014;175(3):584–6.

23. Nizamic T, Murad MH, Allen LA, et al. Ambulatory inotrope infusions in advanced heart failure: a systematic review and meta-analysis. JACC Heart Fail 2018;6(9):757–67.

24. Hernandez GA, Blumer V, Arcay L, et al. Cardiac resynchronization therapy in inotrope-dependent heart failure patients: a systematic review and meta-analysis. JACC Heart Fail 2018;6(9):734–42.

25. Perkiomaki JS, Ruwald A-C, Kutyifa V, et al. Risk factors and the effect of cardiac resynchronization therapy on cardiac and non-cardiac mortality in MADIT-CRT. Europace 2015;17(12):1816–22.

26. Fendler TJ, Nassif ME, Kennedy KF, et al. Global outcome in patients with left ventricular assist devices. Am J Cardiol 2017;119(7):1069–73.

27. Kirklin JK, Naftel DC, Pagani FD, et al. Sixth INTERMACS annual report: a 10,000-patient database. J Heart Lung Transplant 2014;33(6):555–64.

28. McCartney SL, Patel C, Del Rio JM. Long-term outcomes and management of the heart transplant recipient. Best Pract Res Clin Anaesthesiol 2017;31(2): 237–48.

29. Chronic obstructive pulmonary disease among adults—United States. 2011. Available at: https://www.cdc.gov/mmwr/preview/mmwrhtml/mm6146a2.htm?s_cid=mm6146a2_w. Accessed October 7, 2018.

30. Vogelmeier CF, Criner GJ, Martinez FJ, et al. Global strategy for the diagnosis, management, and prevention of chronic obstructive lung disease 2017 report. GOLD executive summary. Am J Respir Crit Care Med 2017;195(5):557–82.

31. NIH Fact Sheets - Chronic Obstructive Pulmonary Disease (COPD). Available at: https://report.nih.gov/nihfactsheets/ViewFactSheet.aspx?csid=77. Accessed October 7, 2018.

32. WHO | Burden of COPD. WHO. Available at: http://www.who.int/respiratory/copd/burden/en/. Accessed October 7, 2018.

33. Croft JB. Urban-rural county and state differences in chronic obstructive pulmonary disease—United States, 2015. MMWR Morb Mortal Wkly Rep 2018;67. https://doi.org/10.15585/mmwr.mm6707a1.

34. Taking her breath away: the rise of COPD in women. 2013. Available at: https://www.lung.org/assets/documents/research/rise-of-copd-in-women-full.pdf.

35. Berman AR. Management of patients with end-stage chronic obstructive pulmonary disease. Prim Care 2011;38(2):277–97.

36. Ford ES, Murphy LB, Khavjou O, et al. Total and state-specific medical and absenteeism costs of COPD among adults aged 18 years in the United States for 2010 and projections through 2020. Chest 2015;147(1):31–45.

37. Kew KM, Dias S, Cates CJ. Long-acting inhaled therapy (beta-agonists, anticholinergics and steroids) for COPD: a network meta-analysis. Cochrane Database Syst Rev 2014;(3):CD010844.

38. Herath SC, Poole P. Prophylactic antibiotic therapy for chronic obstructive pulmonary disease (COPD). Cochrane Database Syst Rev 2013;(11):CD009764.

39. Elkington H, White P, Addington-Hall J, et al. The healthcare needs of chronic obstructive pulmonary disease patients in the last year of life. Palliat Med 2005;19(6):485–91.

40. Brown CE, Engelberg RA, Nielsen EL, et al. Palliative care for patients dying in the intensive care unit with chronic lung disease compared with metastatic cancer. Ann Am Thorac Soc 2016;13(5):684–9.

41. White P, White S, Edmonds P, et al. Palliative care or end-of-life care in advanced chronic obstructive pulmonary disease: a prospective community survey. Br J Gen Pract 2011;61(587):e362–70.

42. Parshall MB, Schwartzstein RM, Adams L, et al. An official American Thoracic Society Statement: update on the mechanisms, assessment, and management of dyspnea. Am J Respir Crit Care Med 2012;185(4):435–52.

43. Kamal AH, Maguire JM, Wheeler JL, et al. Dyspnea review for the palliative care professional: treatment goals and therapeutic options. J Palliat Med 2012;15(1): 106–14.

44. Ahmadi Z, Bernelid E, Currow DC, et al. Prescription of opioids for breathlessness in end-stage COPD: a national population-based study. Int J Chron Obstruct Pulmon Dis 2016;11:2651–7.

45. Rocker G, Young J, Donahue M, et al. Perspectives of patients, family caregivers and physicians about the use of opioids for refractory dyspnea in advanced chronic obstructive pulmonary disease. CMAJ 2012;184(9): E497–504.
46. Simon ST, Higginson IJ, Booth S, et al. Benzodiazepines for the relief of breathlessness in advanced malignant and non-malignant diseases in adults. Cochrane Database Syst Rev 2016;(10):CD007354.
47. Poole P, Chong J, Cates CJ. Mucolytic agents versus placebo for chronic bronchitis or chronic obstructive pulmonary disease. Cochrane Database Syst Rev 2015;(7):CD001287.
48. Molassiotis A, Smith JA, Mazzone P, et al. Symptomatic treatment of cough among adult patients with lung cancer: CHEST guideline and expert panel report. Chest 2017;151(4):861–74.
49. Galbraith S, Fagan P, Perkins P, et al. Does the use of a handheld fan improve chronic dyspnea? A randomized, controlled, crossover trial. J Pain Symptom Manage 2010;39(5):831–8.
50. Cranston JM, Crockett A, Moss J, et al. Domiciliary oxygen for chronic obstructive pulmonary disease. Cochrane Database Syst Rev 2005;(4):CD001744.
51. Continuous or nocturnal oxygen therapy in hypoxemic chronic obstructive lung disease: a clinical trial. Nocturnal Oxygen Therapy Trial Group. Ann Intern Med 1980;93(3):391–8.
52. Chochinov HM, Johnston W, McClement SE, et al. Dignity and distress towards the end of life across four non-cancer populations. PLoS One 2016;11(1). https://doi.org/10.1371/journal.pone.0147607.
53. Spathis A, Booth S. End of life care in chronic obstructive pulmonary disease: in search of a good death. Int J Chron Obstruct Pulmon Dis 2008;3(1):11–29.
54. Puhan MA, Gimeno-Santos E, Cates CJ, et al. Pulmonary rehabilitation following exacerbations of chronic obstructive pulmonary disease. Cochrane Database Syst Rev 2016;(12):CD005305.
55. Carlin BW. Pulmonary rehabilitation and chronic lung disease: opportunities for the respiratory therapist. Respir Care 2009;54(8):1091–9.
56. Stapleton RD, Randall Curtis J. End of life considerations in older patients with lung disease. Clin Chest Med 2007;28(4):801–11, vii.
57. Rocker GM, Simpson AC, Horton R, et al. Opioid therapy for refractory dyspnea in patients with advanced chronic obstructive pulmonary disease: patients' experiences and outcomes. CMAJ Open 2013;1(1):E27–36.
58. Usmani ZA, Carson KV, Cheng JN, et al. Pharmacological interventions for the treatment of anxiety disorders in chronic obstructive pulmonary disease. Cochrane Database Syst Rev 2011;(11):CD008483.
59. Blinderman CD, Homel P, Andrew Billings J, et al. Symptom distress and quality of life in patients with advanced chronic obstructive pulmonary disease. J Pain Symptom Manage 2009;38(1):115–23.
60. van Dam van Isselt EF, Groenewegen-Sipkema KH, Spruit-van Eijk M, et al. Pain in patients with COPD: a systematic review and meta-analysis. BMJ Open 2014; 4(9). https://doi.org/10.1136/bmjopen-2014-005898.
61. Celli BR, Cote CG, Marin JM, et al. The body-mass index, airflow obstruction, dyspnea, and exercise capacity index in chronic obstructive pulmonary disease. N Engl J Med 2004;350(10):1005–12.
62. Almagro P, Soriano JB, Cabrera FJ, et al. Short- and medium-term prognosis in patients hospitalized for COPD exacerbation: the CODEX index. Chest 2014; 145(5):972–80.

63. Criner GJ, Cordova F, Sternberg AL, et al. The national emphysema treatment trial (NETT). Am J Respir Crit Care Med 2011;184(8):881–93.
64. McKenna RJ, Benditt JO, DeCamp M, et al. Safety and efficacy of median sternotomy versus video-assisted thoracic surgery for lung volume reduction surgery. J Thorac Cardiovasc Surg 2004;127(5):1350–60.
65. Meena M, Dixit R, Singh M, et al. Surgical and bronchoscopic lung volume reduction in chronic obstructive pulmonary disease. Pulm Med 2014;2014. https://doi.org/10.1155/2014/757016.
66. Eberhardt R, Gompelmann D, Herth FJ, et al. Endoscopic bronchial valve treatment: patient selection and special considerations. Int J Chron Obstruct Pulmon Dis 2015;10:2147–57.
67. Aziz F, Penupolu S, Xu X, et al. Lung transplant in end-staged chronic obstructive pulmonary disease (COPD) patients: a concise review. J Thorac Dis 2010; 2(2):111–6.
68. Osadnik CR, Tee VS, Carson-Chahhoud KV, et al. Non-invasive ventilation for the management of acute hypercapnic respiratory failure due to exacerbation of chronic obstructive pulmonary disease. Cochrane Database Syst Rev 2017;(7):CD004104.
69. Gadre SK, Duggal A, Mireles-Cabodevila E, et al. Acute respiratory failure requiring mechanical ventilation in severe chronic obstructive pulmonary disease (COPD). Medicine (Baltimore) 2018;97(17). https://doi.org/10.1097/MD. 0000000000010487.
70. Gadre S, Duggal A, Guzman J. Epidemiological characteristics and outcomes of patients with severe COPD requiring mechanical ventilation. Chest 2014; 146(4):58A.
71. Fanelli V, Costamagna A, Ranieri VM. Extracorporeal support for severe acute respiratory failure. Semin Respir Crit Care Med 2014;35(4):519–27.
72. Abrams DC, Brenner K, Burkart KM, et al. Pilot study of extracorporeal carbon dioxide removal to facilitate extubation and ambulation in exacerbations of chronic obstructive pulmonary disease. Ann Am Thorac Soc 2013;10(4):307–14.
73. Hosenpud JD, Bennett LE, Keck BM, et al. Effect of diagnosis on survival benefit of lung transplantation for end-stage lung disease. Lancet 1998; 351(9095):24–7.
74. Lane CR, Tonelli AR. Lung transplantation in chronic obstructive pulmonary disease: patient selection and special considerations. Int J Chron Obstruct Pulmon Dis 2015;10:2137–46.
75. Yusen RD, Edwards LB, Kucheryavaya AY, et al. The Registry of the International Society for Heart and Lung Transplantation: Thirty-First Adult Lung and Heart–Lung Transplant Report—2014; Focus Theme: Retransplantation. J Heart Lung Transplant 2014;33(10):1009–24.
76. Gott M, Gardiner C, Small N, et al. Barriers to advance care planning in chronic obstructive pulmonary disease. Palliat Med 2009;23(7):642–8.
77. Landers A, Wiseman R, Pitama S, et al. Patient perceptions of severe COPD and transitions towards death: a qualitative study identifying milestones and developing key opportunities. NPJ Prim Care Respir Med 2015;25:15043.
78. Snyder JJ, Collins AJ. Association of preventive health care with atherosclerotic heart disease and mortality in CKD. J Am Soc Nephrol 2009;20(7):1614–22.
79. Statistics | The Kidney Project | UCSF. Available at: https://pharm.ucsf.edu/ kidney/need/statistics. Accessed October 29, 2018.
80. Berger TG, Steinhoff M. Pruritus and renal failure. Semin Cutan Med Surg 2011; 30(2):99–100.

81. O'Connor NR, Kumar P. Conservative management of end-stage renal disease without dialysis: a systematic review. J Palliat Med 2012;15(2):228–35.
82. Hemodialysis Adequacy 2006 Work Group. Clinical practice guidelines for hemodialysis adequacy, update 2006. Am J Kidney Dis 2006;48(Suppl 1):S2–90.
83. Moss AH. Revised dialysis clinical practice guideline promotes more informed decision-making. Clin J Am Soc Nephrol 2010;5(12):2380–3.
84. Rayner HC, Zepel L, Fuller DS, et al. Recovery time, quality of life, and mortality in hemodialysis patients: the Dialysis Outcomes and Practice Patterns Study (DOPPS). Am J Kidney Dis 2014;64(1):86–94.
85. Canaud B, Tong L, Tentori F, et al. Clinical practices and outcomes in elderly hemodialysis patients: results from the Dialysis Outcomes and Practice Patterns Study (DOPPS). Clin J Am Soc Nephrol 2011;6(7):1651–62.
86. Johansen KL, Chertow GM, Jin C, et al. Significance of frailty among dialysis patients. J Am Soc Nephrol 2007;18(11):2960–7.
87. Sanchez W, Talwalkar JA. Palliative care for patients with end-stage liver disease ineligible for liver transplantation. Gastroenterol Clin North Am 2006;35(1):201–19.
88. Murphy SL, Xu JQ, Kochanek KD, et al. Deaths: Final data for 2015. National Vital Statistics Reports. Hyattsville, MD: National Center for Health Statistics 2017;66(6):75.
89. Abstracts of the Biennial Meeting of the International Association for the Study of the Liver, April 15-16, 2002 and the 37th Annual Meeting of the European Association for the Study of the Liver, April 18-21, 2002. Madrid, Spain. J Hepatol 2002;36(Suppl 1):1–298.
90. Disease burden in patients with chronic hepatitis C virus (HCV) infection in a United States (US) private health insurance claims database analysis from 2003 to 2010. Available at: http://www.natap.org/2011/AASLD/AASLD_48.htm. Accessed October 29, 2018.
91. Wigg AJ, McCormick R, Wundke R, et al. Efficacy of a chronic disease management model for patients with chronic liver failure. Clin Gastroenterol Hepatol 2013;11(7):850–8.e1-4.
92. Vilstrup H, Amodio P, Bajaj J, et al. Hepatic encephalopathy in chronic liver disease: 2014 Practice Guideline by the American Association for the Study of Liver Diseases and the European Association for the Study of the Liver. Hepatology 2014;60(2):715–35.
93. Sharma P, Sharma BC. Disaccharides in the treatment of hepatic encephalopathy. Metab Brain Dis 2013;28(2):313–20.
94. Pérez-Ayuso RM, Arroyo V, Planas R, et al. Randomized comparative study of efficacy of furosemide versus spironolactone in nonazotemic cirrhosis with ascites. Relationship between the diuretic response and the activity of the renin-aldosterone system. Gastroenterology 1983;84(5 Pt 1):961–8.
95. The serum-ascites albumin gradient is superior to the exudate-transudate concept in the differential diagnosis of ascites. Available at: https://www.ncbi.nlm.nih.gov/pubmed?term=1616215. Accessed October 29, 2018.
96. Bhalerao A, Mannu GS. Management of pruritus in chronic liver disease. Dermatol Res Pract 2015. https://doi.org/10.1155/2015/295891.
97. Biggins SW, Bambha K. MELD-based liver allocation: who is underserved? Semin Liver Dis 2006;26(3):211–20.
98. Grgurevic I, Bozin T, Madir A. Hepatitis C is now curable, but what happens with cirrhosis and portal hypertension afterwards? Clin Exp Hepatol 2017;3(4):181–6.

99. Boyer TD, Haskal ZJ, American Association for the Study of Liver Diseases. The role of transjugular intrahepatic portosystemic shunt (TIPS) in the management of portal hypertension: update 2009. Hepatology 2010;51(1):306.

100. Potosek J, Curry M, Buss M, et al. Integration of palliative care in end-stage liver disease and liver transplantation. J Palliat Med 2014;17(11):1271–7.

101. Wolff B, Machill K, Schumacher D, et al. MARS dialysis in decompensated alcoholic liver disease: a single-center experience. Liver Transpl 2007;13(8): 1189–92.

102. Hanish SI, Stein DM, Scalea JR, et al. Molecular adsorbent recirculating system effectively replaces hepatic function in severe acute liver failure. Ann Surg 2017; 266(4):677–84.

103. Adams CE, Bader J, Horn KV. Timing of hospice referral: assessing satisfaction while the patient receives hospice services. Home Health Care Manag Pract 2009;21(2):109.

Palliative Care in the Management of Human Immunodeficiency Virus/Acquired Immunodeficiency Syndrome in the Primary Care Setting

Linda R. Mitchell, MD[a],*, Nidhi Shah, MD[a], Peter A. Selwyn, MD, MPH[b]

KEYWORDS

• HIV/AIDS • Palliative care • Malignancies • Aging population

KEY POINTS

- Human immunodeficiency virus (HIV) remains particularly prevalent among specific groups, including the younger population and men who have sex with men.
- The disease course is influenced by the presence of other health comorbidities, age, presence of opportunistic infections, non–AIDS-defining illness, functional status, CD4 counts, adherence to highly active antiretroviral treatment (HAART), and viral load on HAART.
- HIV+ individuals have a high risk of developing several AIDS-defining conditions (ADCs). As they become older adults, they are more likely to die from non-ADCs than ADCs.
- The use of palliative care in HIV is important to address early advance care planning, offer emotional and psychosocial support, and provide pain and symptom management, especially at end of life.

INTRODUCTION

In the early days of human immunodeficiency virus (HIV) and acquired immunodeficiency syndrome (AIDS), patients and clinicians came to know about the infection as a terminal condition. Introduction of highly active antiretroviral treatment (HAART) in the mid-1990s transformed the disease trajectory for many patients with HIV/

Disclosure Statement: The authors have nothing to disclose.
[a] Palliative Medicine Program, Department of Family and Social Medicine, Montefiore Medical Center, The University Hospital for the Albert Einstein College of Medicine, 3347 Steuben Avenue, Bronx, NY 10467, USA; [b] Department of Family and Social Medicine, Palliative Medicine Program, Montefiore Medical Center, The University Hospital for the Albert Einstein College of Medicine, 3544 Jerome Avenue, Bronx, NY 10467, USA
* Corresponding author.
E-mail address: lesteban@montefiore.org

Prim Care Clin Office Pract 46 (2019) 433–445
https://doi.org/10.1016/j.pop.2019.05.009
0095-4543/19/© 2019 Elsevier Inc. All rights reserved.

primarycare.theclinics.com

AIDS and transitioned the course from a terminal disease to a chronic disease model. The changing nature of disease management coupled with the evolution of palliative care, demands that primary care clinicians master the skills of primary palliative care in this subset of patients to provide highest quality of life and best care coordination.

The evolving role of palliative care for HIV as a chronic illness stems from many factors, as illustrated in **Fig. 1**. The post-HAART era has seen a dramatic decline in the rates of AIDS-defining opportunistic infections (OIs) among HIV-infected patients. Progression to AIDS is still prevalent and thus this topic deserves a review of the unique elements of late-stage AIDS, AIDS-defining illnesses, non–AIDS-defining malignancies, as well as the incorporation of palliative care services to improve quality of life for these patients.

Ultimately, advance care planning (ACP) and end-of-life issues have become more challenging and complex due to the transition of HIV/AIDS to a chronic condition, compared with the uniform, rapid, and predictable course it previously took. This article reviews the epidemiology of HIV/AIDS, prognostic indicators, frailty, OIs, specific AIDS-defining malignancies and non–AIDS-defining malignancies, role of palliative care, ACP, and the role of HAART in patients dying of late-stage AIDS.

Epidemiology

In nearly 4 decades since the first AIDS cases were identified, the epidemiology of HIV/AIDS has transformed in many ways. According to the most recent Centers for Disease Control and Prevention (CDC) HIV/AIDS Surveillance Report,

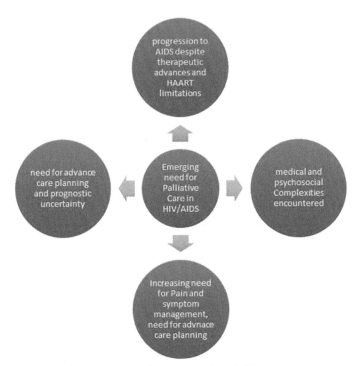

Fig. 1. Evolving role of palliative care for HIV as a chronic illness.

approximately 1.2 million people in the United States have been diagnosed with AIDS since the early 1980s. Between 1987, the first year HIV was listed as a cause of death on a death certificate, and 2015, more than half a million people died due to HIV disease.[1] Despite gains in life expectancy, HIV continues to be the ninth leading cause of death among adults aged 25 to 44. As of January 2016, approximately 1.1 million people are living with HIV/AIDS in the United States. This is especially true among young adults and adolescents ages 13 to 24, of which 51% did not know they were infected.[1]

The landscape of demographic prevalence is changing rapidly, with newly diagnosed HIV/AIDS being most significant among young adults (20–39 years), with the chronic nature of the disease impacting the older population, with adults older than 50 representing approximately 50% of HIV-infected individuals.

Gay and bisexual men or men who have sex with men (MSM) (82%) remain the highest risk population to be affected by HIV. In this population, overall HIV diagnosis from 2011 to 2015 has remained stable. Black/African American gay and bisexual men are affected by HIV more than any other group. In addition, black transgender women have the highest percentage among all transgender women living with HIV.[1]

Prognostic Indicators

Prognostication, or the ability to predict the course of a disease, is critical to the care of patients with HIV/AIDS. In the pre-HAART era, a patient's prognosis could largely be predicted based on viral load and CD4 cell count. Estimates of life expectancy were less than 1 year in some US cohorts.[2] In the post-HAART era, mortality rates for individuals infected and treated with HAART are now closer to the general population, with an estimated mean survival of 35 years.[3] Beyond the introduction of HAART, the disease course is influenced by a variety of factors, including the presence of other medical comorbidities, age, presence of OIs, non–AIDS-defining illnesses, functional status, CD4 cell count, adherence to HAART therapy, and viral load once on HAART. One key factor consistently shown to correlate with poor prognosis is failure of the patient to seek antiretroviral treatment.

Primary care providers are advised to seek counsel of expert HIV physicians and palliative care providers for patients presenting with findings consistent with late-stage HIV. In addition, the antiretroviral therapy cohort collaboration has created 2 risk calculators for those who are older than 16, have not previously been treated with HAART, and are infected with HIV-1. These calculators can be found at the University of Bristol Web site (http://www.bristol.ac.uk/art-cc/research/calculator/).

The Centers for Medicare and Medicaid Services (CMS) local coverage determinations (LCDs) assist with the identification of a Medicare beneficiary who may be eligible for hospice services. Patients with terminal disease with life expectancy of 6 months or less, if it takes the natural course, are eligible for hospice services. The LCDs are not strict criteria, but rather guidelines. It is important to become familiar with these guidelines and consult with specialists for further guidance. The content in **Box 1** partially entails the HIV/AIDS-related LCDs current as of this article's publication.

Frailty

As HIV-infected individuals age into the geriatric population, they are faced with higher rates of comorbid illnesses and multimorbidity. These illnesses include liver disease, cardiovascular disease, kidney impairment, cancers, osteoporosis, cognitive decline,

---

Box 1

Human immunodeficiency virus/acquired immunodeficiency syndrome (HIV/AIDS)-related local coverage determinations

Patients will be considered to be in the terminal stage of their illness (life expectancy of 6 months or less) if they meet the following criteria:

HIV disease (1 and 2 must be present; factors from 3 will add supporting documentation)

1. CD4+ count less than 25 cells/μL or persistent viral load greater than 100,000 copies/mL, plus *1* of the following:
   a. Central nervous system lymphoma
   b. Untreated, or not responsive to treatment, wasting (loss of 33% lean body mass)
   c. Mycobacterium avium complex (MAC) bacteremia, untreated, unresponsive to treatment, or treatment refused
   d. Progressive multifocal leukoencephalopathy
   e. Systemic lymphoma, with advanced HIV disease and partial response to chemotherapy
   f. Visceral Kaposi sarcoma unresponsive to therapy
   g. Renal failure in the absence of dialysis
   h. Cryptosporidium infection
   i. Toxoplasmosis, unresponsive to therapy

2. Decreased performance status, as measured by the Karnofsky Performance Status scale, of ≤50

3. Documentation of the following factors will support eligibility for hospice care:
   a. Chronic persistent diarrhea for 1 year
   b. Persistent serum albumin less than 2.5
   c. Concomitant, active substance abuse
   d. Age older than 50 years
   e. Absence of antiretroviral, chemotherapeutic, and prophylactic drug therapy related specifically to HIV disease
   f. Advanced AIDS dementia complex
   g. Toxoplasmosis
   h. Congestive heart failure, symptomatic at rest

Data from CMS. LCD for hospice determining terminal status. Available at: www.cms.gov.

---

and frailty. Aging individuals with HIV and multimorbidity are at an increased risk for polypharmacy.[4]

Frailty, as referred to in HIV literature, is defined as decreased ability to recover from additional injury and includes wasting, slowing, and weakness characterized by the frailty phenotype and the frailty-related phenotype.[5] The most clinically useful tool to assess frailty and functional capacity is the Veterans Aging Cohort Study (VACS) index, which combines clinical measures of immunodeficiency, viral load, and organ system compromise to estimate the risk of morbidity and mortality.[6]

Individuals aging with HIV also tend to have a low or poor social support systems, which may translate into more frequent hospitalizations and overall mortality.[7]

Opportunistic Infections

On June 5, 1981, the CDC reported 5 cases of pneumocystis pneumonia (PCP), among previously health young men in Los Angeles.[8] These cases would later be identified as the first documented cases of AIDS in the United States, and PCP would be labeled an OI and 1 of the 26 AIDS-defining illnesses. For the scope of this article, 5 frequently diagnosed AIDS-related OIs according to the National Institutes of Health Guidelines for Prevention and Treatment of Opportunistic Infections[9] in conjunction with a more recent 2015 study conducted in San Francisco that investigated the most common OIs among more than 20,000 individuals from 1981 to 2012[10] are listed (**Table 1**).

Acquired Immunodeficiency Syndrome–Defining and Non–Acquired Immunodeficiency Syndrome–Defining Malignancies

Patients infected with HIV have a high risk of developing several forms of cancer. These malignancies may arise when the immune system is damaged and CD4 T-cell count is low. Virally induced neoplasia, such as Kaposi sarcoma (associated with human herpes virus 8 [HHV8]), cervical cancer (associated with human papilloma virus [HPV]), and aggressive non-Hodgkin (NHL) lymphoma

Table 1
Opportunistic infections (OIs) with clinical presentation, specifics for diagnosis, and treatment

Type of OI	Common Clinical Presentation	Specifics for Diagnosis Modality	Treatment/Primary Prophylaxis
Pneumocystis pneumonia (PCP)	Subacute onset of dyspnea, fever, nonproductive cough and chest discomfort, oral thrush (common coinfection), spontaneous pneumothorax.	Histopathologic or cytopathologic demonstration of organisms in tissue, bronchoalveolar lavage (BAL) fluid, or induced sputum samples.[11] An alternative method for diagnosing PCP is polymerase chain reaction (PCR).[12]	Highly active antiretroviral treatment combined with chemoprophylaxis in patients with CD4 Cells <200 cells/ mm^3; Bactrim remains treatment of choice.
Disseminated *Mycobacterium avium* complex (MAC) disease	Fever, weight loss, night sweats, fatigue, diarrhea, lymphadenopathy, hepatosplenomegaly, anemia, and elevated values of liver tests.	Clinical signs and isolation of MAC from cultures of bodily fluids.	CD4 counts <50 cells/mm^3 Azithromycin and clarithromycin are preferred.
Toxoplasmosis gondii encephalitis	Focal encephalitis with headache, fever, confusion, and motor weakness.	Seropositive for immunoglobulin antibodies.	CD4 counts <100 cells/ mm^3 combination of pyrimethamine, sulfadiazine and leucovorin.
Cytomegalovirus (CMV)	Retinitis ± floaters, scotomata or peripheral visual field defects.	Detected by PCR, antigen assays or culture.	Using antiretroviral therapy to keep CD4 count >100 cells/ mm^3.
Cryptococcal meningitis	Fever, headache, and general malaise manifesting as subacute meningitis and can disseminate to nearly any organ.	Cerebrospinal fluid with mildly elevate serum protein, low to normal glucose and lymphocytes. India Ink stain.	Consists of 3 phases: induction, consolidation, and maintenance. Start with Amphotericin B and flucytosine for 2 wk.

(associated with Epstein-Barr virus [EBV]) have been defined as AIDS-defining cancers (ADCs).

Non-ADCs (NADCs) are an increasing cause of morbidity and mortality in HIV-infected individuals, especially in the aging population, and include Hodgkin lymphoma and cancers of the mouth, throat, liver, lung, and anus. In a retrospective review from 1996 to 2006, the proportion of deaths from NADCs increased from 7.3% to 15.4%, whereas the ADCs decreased.[13]

As with opportunistic infections, the introduction of combination antiretroviral therapy (cART) in 1996 has decreased the incidence of AIDS-related malignances and increased the incidence of non–AIDS-defining malignances by threefold.[14,15] Introduction of HAART has decreased the risk of developing Kaposi sarcoma (KS) and NHL, in contrast to invasive cervical cancers.[16,17]

The following sections examine the most relevant cancers, focusing on epidemiologic trends, presentation, progression, and treatment improvements.

ACQUIRED IMMUNODEFICIENCY SYNDROME–DEFINING MALIGNANCIES
Kaposi Sarcoma

KS is a hypervascular disease that most commonly affects the skin, intestinal tracts, and lungs. Among the general population, it is a rare form of cancer, yet in the HIV-infected population, KS is the most common AIDS-associated malignancy. With the availability of HAART, incidence of KS has been drastically reduced. Although 5-year survival from diagnosis data indicate a significant improvement from 10% pre-HAART to 73% post-HAART, the natural history of KS continues to create significant morbidity and mortality.[18,19] A 15-point prognostic index has been developed by researchers that attempts to categorize patients into prognostic tiers of best, intermediate, and worst prognosis based on age, occurrence of KS at or after AIDS onset, presence of comorbid conditions, and CD4 cell count.[20] Treatment strategies are advised per prognostic tier, with HAART alone being recommended for the "best" tier, and HAART with systemic chemotherapy being the treatment of choice for the "worst" tier, enabling a median survival of 242 days.

Non-Hodgkin lymphoma

HIV-infected individuals have greatly elevated risk of NHL, particularly the AIDS-defining NHL subtypes: diffuse large B-cell lymphoma, Burkitt lymphoma, and primary lymphomas arising in the central nervous system. In-depth discussion of these cancers is beyond the scope of this article.

HAART has reduced the incidence of NHL, but it remains the second most common AIDS-associated malignancy worldwide. Dramatic declines in KS and NHL have been attributed to improved immune control of oncogenic viruses with HIV treatment.[21] Multiple studies have demonstrated considerable elevation in risk for AIDS-defining NHL subtypes in the HAART era in those with AIDS compared with those with HIV-only, which supports severity of immune deficiency as a primary determinant of risk for these subtypes.[22]

Although NHL consists of an array of lymphocyte blood tumors, 95% of AIDS-related lymphomas are derived from B cells. Compared with NHL encountered in the HIV-negative population, HIV-infected populations present with advanced diseases, B symptoms, extranodal disease, leptomeningeal disease, and disease in unusual locations.[23] Non-Hodgkin lymphoma has lower survival rates than patients with other AIDS-defining malignancies, such as KS or cervical cancer (10-year survival: 48.2% $\pm$ 4.3% vs 72.8% $\pm$ 4.0% vs 78.5% $\pm$ 9.9%; P <.001).[19]

Invasive cervical carcinoma
Persistent oncogenic HPV infection with low CD counts remains the major risk factor for cervical cancer. Women living with HIV have been found to be 8 times more likely to develop invasive ADC of the cervix than women who were not HIV infected.[24] A large multicenter collaborative prospective study found HIV-infected women with baseline CD4+ T cells of $\geq$350, 200 to 349, and fewer than 200 cells/μL had a 2.3-times, 3.0-times, and 7.7-times increase in incidence of invasive cervical carcinoma (ICC), respectively, compared with HIV-uninfected women,[25] most likely due to the disease becoming a chronic illness leading to persistent HPV infection. Median survival is up to age 73.9 years in a 25-year-old woman with HIV and ICC with management of chronic HPV infection and ICC.[26] Overall, greater surveillance and treatment of these types of cancers are needed, especially given the substantially higher risk compared with general population.

Non–AIDS-DEFINING MALIGNANCIES
Anal Cancer

In United States, the rates of anal cancer among MSM and immunosuppressed men now exceed the rates of cervical cancer among women.[27] In the NA-ACCORD study, HIV-infected MSM experienced the greatest risk for anal cancer with incidence rates greater than 80 times as high as HIV-uninfected individuals. Data regarding the impact of HAART on incidence of anal cancer is controversial, suggesting increased survival in the post-HAART era leads to longer exposure to HPV infection, thus increasing incidence of anal cancer.[28] There is a need for further studies on preventive strategies for anal cancer in this patient population.

Head and Neck Cancer

Oral HPV infection, in additional to tobacco and alcohol exposure, has been recently noted to be an important cause of head and neck cancers.[29] The risk in HIV-infected individuals is twofold higher than in the general population, and risk stratification based on anatomic site reveals a sixfold increase in risk of HPV-related tonsillar squamous cell carcinoma.[30] HAART does not appear to reconstitute HPV-specific immunity, as some reduction in risk for oropharyngeal cancer in the post-HAART era has been reported,[31] but not consistently.[24,32]

Hepatocellular Cancer

Persons infected with HIV, especially injecting drug users, have a greatly increased incidence of hepatitis B virus (HBV) and hepatitis C virus (HCV) infection compared with the general population, and consequently are at a greater risk for hepatocellular carcinoma (HCC).[33,34] In the era of HAART, coinfected patients have not necessarily experienced higher incidence of HCC than among mono-infected patients as compared with increased risk of cirrhosis and liver-related deaths.[35,36] All HIV-infected patients should be screened for HBV with hepatitis B surface antigen, anti-HBs, and hepatitis B core antibody. Individuals without immunity to HBV should be vaccinated; however, response to vaccination is poor, especially in patients whose CD4 cell count is <200 cells/mm^3. The American Association for the Study of Liver Disease recommends screening these patients every 6 to 12 months with alpha-fetoprotein measurement and imaging. Although separate recommendations for HIV-HCV coinfection do not exist, screening remains important in this population, as HCC incidence has been increasing among HIV-infected individuals. HAART and better HCV treatments may be associated with a decreased risk of hepatic decompensation and increased survival of coinfected patients with cirrhosis, leading to increased incidence of HCC.[28]

Lung Cancer

Lung cancer is a leading non–AIDS-defining cancer and is the most frequent cause of cancer deaths in HIV-infected persons. This is most likely due to higher smoking rates among HIV-infected persons, but also due to independent, HIV-related increased lung cancer risk. With improved HIV disease control, larger numbers of patients are surviving long enough to develop and die from lung cancer.

Prognosis of HIV-infected persons with lung cancer is worse than uninfected persons in several studies, but it is not known if this is related to treatment disparities, lung cancer therapy intolerance, greater risk of treatment toxicity, or competing risk from AIDS and non–AIDS-related morbidity. Last, lung cancer prevention and early detection, an area of major clinical interest in HIV-uninfected persons, is still an emerging area of study for HIV-infected persons.[37–40]

Hodgkin Lymphoma

Hodgkin lymphoma (HL) has increased 10-fold in individuals with HIV infection.[33] HL incidence is greatest with moderate immunosuppression, and improvements in CD4 lymphocyte counts resulting from combination antiretroviral therapy might explain the apparent increase in HL.[41] However, it is interesting that the incidence of HL has not decreased in the HAART era, and in fact, 2 large studies in the United States have reported increasing rates.[17,31,41] Both HL and NHL appear to develop from B-lymphocyte transformation. Therefore, EBV-associated subsets of HL may be associated with immune dysfunction through similar mechanisms underlying the association with NHL.[42]

Colorectal, Breast, and Prostate Cancer

Screening for HIV-infected individuals for colorectal and breast cancer should follow the guidelines for the general population, as there is no clear evidence that the incidence of these cancers are higher in patients with HIV. The incidence rate of prostate cancer in HIV-positive persons is lower than HIV-negative persons.[43] Screening for HIV-positive persons for prostate cancer remains controversial, just as in the general population, because of differing recommendations from the US Preventive Services Task Force and American Urologic Association. As with the general population, there is an increased rate of these cancers with aging individuals with HIV.

Palliative care for patients with human immunodeficiency virus/acquired immunodeficiency syndrome

Palliative care is a medical subspecialty that focuses on preventing and relieving suffering, as well as providing the best possible quality of life for patients, and their families, facing serious illnesses. With HIV becoming a chronic illness in the HAART era and patients continuing to advance to AIDS despite therapeutic advances, the need for palliative care intervention for management of pain and symptom burden, alleviating psychosocial distress, early ACP, and excellent end-of-life care is crucial. The little literature that exists on the contemporary state of palliative care in HIV infection points to underutilization of hospice and palliative care in this population. It is likely that palliative care intervention could improve HIV outcomes, through better adherence to HAART, retention in HIV primary care, and virologic suppression.[44]

Patients with HIV share a high degree of comorbidity and multimorbidity, including higher than average rates of age-related comorbidities, such as hypertension, diabetes mellitus, renal failure, cardiovascular disease, liver disease, and neurocognitive impairment.[45] Some of the challenges faced by primary care providers in caring for patients with HIV/AIDS include the highly variable prognostic course of the illness, immunologic response to HAART, response to therapy for OI, and presence of malignancy. The authors were unable to find a standard prognostic tool, although the most commonly used is the VACS index developed by the National Institute of Medicine. The tool combines 7 variables to predict mortality in HIV-infected individuals: age, CD4 cell count, HIV viral load, hemoglobin, Fibrosis-4 Index, presence of hepatitis C, and glomerular filtration rate.[6,46]

Pain and Symptom Management

Pain remains the most common reason for referral to palliative care in the outpatient setting, reported in 90% of cases, with chronic pain experienced by two-thirds of the population. Other symptoms include depression (48%), anxiety (21%), insomnia (30%), and constipation (32%).[47] Pain is most likely neuropathic, but also could be musculoskeletal, with back pain being the most commonly reported type.[48] Presence of chronic pain in this population leads to functional impairment 10 times more often than in the general population.

Nonpain Symptoms

Reported nonpain psychosocial symptoms include worrying, feeling sad, difficulty sleeping, feeling irritable, feeling nervous, and difficulty concentrating. Nonpain physical symptoms reported by patients include fatigue, drowsiness, sweats, cough, dry mouth, diarrhea, dyspnea, pruritus, anorexia, loss of interest in sexual activity, and nausea.

Advance Care Planning

ACP is defined as a process of making decisions about the care a patient would want to receive if the patient became unable to speak for himself or herself. These are the patient's decisions to make, regardless of what he or she chose for care, and the decisions are based on personal values, preferences, and discussions with loved ones. A study published in 1993, during the era of mono/dual antiretroviral treatment, stressed the importance of HIV-infected individuals completing advance directives (ADs). At that time, their disease would progress rapidly, leaving them unable to make medical decisions for themselves.[49] The studies conducted in the post-HAART era show increased rate of AD completion but no improvement of patient satisfaction with health care.[50] The FAmily CEntered (FACE) ACP study provides more insights into ACP in this vulnerable patient population and identifies barriers to ACP in this patient population and can serve as a valuable resource for the primary care clinics.[51]

Discontinuation of Highly Active Anti-Retroviral Treatment in the Patient Dying of Late-Stage Acquired Immunodeficiency Syndrome

Discontinuation of HAART may result in a variety of clinical outcomes that would typically be considered undesirable, such as viral rebound, immune decompensation, and disease advancement. Therefore, in patients who are clinically stable with good immune status and adequate viral load suppression, discontinuation of HAART is not recommended. Decisions to continue or discontinue HAART should involve the patient-caregiver dyads at end of life. Clinical criteria for withdrawal of HAART at end of life do not exist. The potential theoretic benefits of continuing HAART include suppression of more pathogenic virus, protection against HIV encephalopathy/dementia, relief of constitutional symptoms associated with high viral load, and the psychological comfort of combatting the disease felt by some patients on HAART. Alternatively, potential risks or certain reasons to consider stopping HAART include toxicity or pharmacologic interventions with comfort medications, diminished quality of life return versus treatment burden, therapeutic confusion, and distraction from end-of-life or ACP.

REFERENCES

1. Centers for Disease Control and Prevention. HIV/AIDS Surveillance Report. 2016. Available at: http://www.cdc.gov/hiv/topics/surveillance/resources/reports/. Accessed September 20, 2018.
2. Lemp GF, Payne SF, Neal D, et al. Survival trends for patients with AIDS. JAMA 1990;263(3):402–6.
3. Lohse N, Hansen AB, Pedersen G, et al. Survival of persons with and without HIV infection in Denmark, 1995-2005. Ann Intern Med 2007;146(2):87–95.
4. Smith JM, Flexner C. The challenge of polypharmacy in an aging population and implications for future antiretroviral therapy development. AIDS 2017;31(Suppl 2): S173–84.
5. Desquilbet L, Margolick JB, Fried LP, et al. Relationship between a frailty-related phenotype and progressive deterioration of the immune system in HIV-infected men. J Acquir Immune Defic Syndr 2009;50(3):299–306.
6. Justice AC, Modur SP, Tate JP, et al. Predictive accuracy of the Veterans Aging Cohort Study index for mortality with HIV infection: a North American cross cohort analysis. J Acquir Immune Defic Syndr 2013;62(2):149–63.
7. Greysen SR, Horwitz LI, Covinsky KE, et al. Does social isolation predict hospitalization and mortality among HIV+ and uninfected older veterans? J Am Geriatr Soc 2013;61(9):1456–63.
8. Centers for Disease Control (CDC). Pneumocystis pneumonia—Los Angeles. MMWR Morb Mortal Wkly Rep 1981;30:250–2.
9. Panel on opportunistic infections in HIV-infected adults and adolescents. Guidelines for the prevention and treatment of opportunistic infections in HIV-infected adults and adolescents: recommendations from the Centers for Disease Control and Prevention, the National Institutes of Health, and the HIV Medicine Association of the Infectious Diseases Society of America. Available at: https://aidsinfo.nih.gov/contentfiles/lvguidelines/adult_oi.pdf. Accessed September 18, 2018.
10. Djawe K, Buchacz K, Hsu L, et al. Mortality risk after AIDS-defining opportunistic illness among HIV-infected persons–San Francisco, 1981-2012. J Infect Dis 2015; 212(9):1366–75.
11. Hidalgo A, Falcó V, Mauleón S, et al. Accuracy of high-resolution CT in distinguishing between *Pneumocystis carinii* pneumonia and non-*Pneumocystis carinii* pneumonia in AIDS patients. Eur Radiol 2003;13(5):1179–84.
12. Roger PM, Vandenbos F, Pugliese P, et al. Persistence of *Pneumocystis carinii* after effective treatment of *P. carinii* pneumonia is not related to relapse or survival among patients infected with human immunodeficiency virus. Clin Infect Dis 1998;26(2):509–10.

13. Antiretroviral Therapy Cohort Collaboration. Causes of death in HIV-1-infected patients treated with antiretroviral therapy, 1996-2006: collaborative analysis of 13 HIV cohort studies. Clin Infect Dis 2010;50(10):1387–96.

14. Yanik EL, Napravnik S, Cole SR, et al. Incidence and timing of cancer in HIV-infected individuals following initiation of combination antiretroviral therapy. Clin Infect Dis 2013;57(5):756–64.

15. Cancer in HIV and aging 2017; Available from: http://hiv-age.org/2017/08/17/cancer-hiv-aging-2/.

16. Cobucci RN, Lima PH, de Souza PC, et al. Assessing the impact of HAART on the incidence of defining and non-defining AIDS cancers among patients with HIV/AIDS: a systematic review. J Infect Public Health 2015;8(1):1–10.

17. Engels EA, Pfeiffer RM, Goedert JJ, et al. Trends in cancer risk among people with AIDS in the United States 1980-2002. AIDS 2006;20(12):1645–54.

18. HIV/AIDS- Related Cancer: Statistics 2018; Available from: https://www.cancer.net/cancer-types/hivaids-related-cancer/statstics. Accessed June.

19. Gotti D, Raffetti E, Albini L, et al. Survival in HIV-infected patients after a cancer diagnosis in the cART Era: results of an Italian multicenter study. PLoS One 2014; 9(4):e94768.

20. Stebbing J, Sanitt A, Nelson M, et al. A prognostic index for AIDS-associated Kaposi's sarcoma in the era of highly active antiretroviral therapy. Lancet 2006; 367(9521):1495–502.

21. Robbins HA, Shiels MS, Pfeiffer RM, et al. Epidemiologic contributions to recent cancer trends among HIV-infected people in the United States. AIDS 2014;28(6): 881–90.

22. Gibson TM, Morton LM, Shiels MS, et al. Risk of non-Hodgkin lymphoma subtypes in HIV-infected people during the HAART era: a population-based study. AIDS 2014;28(15):2313–8.

23. Cheung MC, Pantanowitz L, Dezube BJ. AIDS-related malignancies: emerging challenges in the era of highly active antiretroviral therapy. Oncologist 2005; 10(6):412–26.

24. Clifford GM, Polesel J, Rickenbach M, et al. Cancer risk in the Swiss HIV Cohort Study: associations with immunodeficiency, smoking, and highly active antiretroviral therapy. J Natl Cancer Inst 2005;97(6):425–32.

25. Abraham AG, D'Souza G, Jing Y, et al. Invasive cervical cancer risk among HIV-infected women: a North American multicohort collaboration prospective study. J Acquir Immune Defic Syndr 2013;62(4):405–13.

26. Ghebre RG, Grover S, Xu MJ, et al. Cervical cancer control in HIV-infected women: Past, present and future. Gynecol Oncol Rep 2017;21:101–8.

27. Palefsky J. Human papillomavirus and anal neoplasia. Curr HIV/AIDS Rep 2008; 5(2):78–85.

28. Wang CC, Silverberg MJ, Abrams DI. Non-AIDS-defining malignancies in the HIV-infected population. Curr Infect Dis Rep 2014;16(6):406.

29. IARC Working Group on the Evaluation of Carcinogenic Risks to Humans. Human papillomaviruses. IARC Monogr Eval Carcinog Risks Hum 2007;90:1–636.

30. Frisch M, Biggar RJ, Engels EA, et al. Association of cancer with AIDS-related immunosuppression in adults. JAMA 2001;285(13):1736–45.

31. Engels EA, Biggar RJ, Hall HI, et al. Cancer risk in people infected with human immunodeficiency virus in the United States. Int J Cancer 2008;123(1): 187–94.

32. Powles T, Robinson D, Stebbing J, et al. Highly active antiretroviral therapy and the incidence of non-AIDS-defining cancers in people with HIV infection. J Clin Oncol 2009;27(6):884–90.

33. Grulich AE, van Leeuwen MT, Falster MO, et al. Incidence of cancers in people with HIV/AIDS compared with immunosuppressed transplant recipients: a meta-analysis. Lancet 2007;370(9581):59–67.

34. McGinnis KA, Fultz SL, Skanderson M, et al. Hepatocellular carcinoma and non-Hodgkin's lymphoma: the roles of HIV, hepatitis C infection, and alcohol abuse. J Clin Oncol 2006;24(31):5005–9.

35. Kramer JR, Giordano TP, Souchek J, et al. The effect of HIV coinfection on the risk of cirrhosis and hepatocellular carcinoma in U.S. veterans with hepatitis C. Am J Gastroenterol 2005;100(1):56–63.

36. Di Benedetto N, Peralta M, Alvarez E, et al. Incidence of hepatocellular carcinoma in hepatitis C cirrhotic patients with and without HIV infection: a cohort study, 1999-2011. Ann Hepatol 2013;13(1):38–44.

37. Sigel K, Makinson A, Thaler J. Lung cancer in persons with HIV. Curr Opin HIV AIDS 2017;12(1):31–8.

38. Makinson A, Tenon JC, Eymard-Duvernay S, et al. Human immunodeficiency virus infection and non-small cell lung cancer: survival and toxicity of antineoplastic chemotherapy in a cohort study. J Thorac Oncol 2011;6(6):1022–9.

39. Suneja G, Lin CC, Simard EP, et al. Disparities in cancer treatment among patients infected with the human immunodeficiency virus. Cancer 2016;122(15): 2399–407.

40. Bearz A, Vaccher E, Martellotta F, et al. Lung cancer in HIV positive patients: the GICAT experience. Eur Rev Med Pharmacol Sci 2014;18(4):500–8.

41. Biggar RJ, Jaffe ES, Goedert JJ, et al. Hodgkin lymphoma and immunodeficiency in persons with HIV/AIDS. Blood 2006;108(12):3786–91.

42. Martis N, Mounier N. Hodgkin lymphoma in patients with HIV infection: a review. Curr Hematol Malig Rep 2012;7(3):228–34.

43. Marcus JL, Chao CR, Leyden WA, et al. Prostate cancer incidence and prostate-specific antigen testing among HIV-positive and HIV-negative men. J Acquir Immune Defic Syndr 2014;66(5):495–502.

44. Harding R, Simms V, Alexander C, et al. Can palliative care integrated within HIV outpatient settings improve pain and symptom control in a low-income country? A prospective, longitudinal, controlled intervention evaluation. AIDS Care 2013; 25(7):795–804.

45. Valderas JM, Starfield B, Sibbald B, et al. Defining comorbidity: implications for understanding health and health services. Ann Fam Med 2009;7(4): 357–63.

46. Vallet-Pichard A, Mallet V, Nalpas B, et al. FIB-4: an inexpensive and accurate marker of fibrosis in HCV infection. comparison with liver biopsy and fibrotest. Hepatology 2007;46(1):32–6.

47. Perry BA, Westfall AO, Molony E, et al. Characteristics of an ambulatory palliative care clinic for HIV-infected patients. J Palliat Med 2013;16(8):934–7.

48. Merlin JS, Walcott M, Ritchie C, et al. 'Two pains together': patient perspectives on psychological aspects of chronic pain while living with HIV. PLoS One 2014; 9(11):e111765.

49. Wachter RM, Lo B. Advance directives for patients with human immunodeficiency virus infection. Crit Care Clin 1993;9(1):125–36.

50. Ho VW, Thiel EC, Rubin HR, et al. The effect of advance care planning on completion of advance directives and patient satisfaction in people with HIV/AIDS. AIDS Care 2000;12(1):97–108.
51. Kimmel AL, Wang J, Scott RK, et al. FAmily CEntered (FACE) advance care planning: study design and methods for a patient-centered communication and decision-making intervention for patients with HIV/AIDS and their surrogate decision-makers. Contemp Clin Trials 2015;43:172–8.

Geriatric Palliative Care

Andy Lazris, MD, CMD

KEYWORDS

- Geriatrics • Geriatric palliative care • Dementia • Parkinson disease • Frailty
- FAST scale • Polypharmacy • Slow medicine

KEY POINTS

- There are limited data that aggressive medical interventions are effective in the geriatric population, especially in those with high frailty scores.
- Palliative care in the elderly is primary care based and seeks to preserve function, reduce discomfort, and enable independence as people age.
- Many conditions, such as dementia, Parkinson, arthritis, pneumonia, and congestive heart failure, have better outcomes when treated with a palliative approach.
- Specific goals of a palliative approach are to reduce polypharmacy, reduce fall risk, prevent hospitalization, and treat patients without focusing on numbers.

In discussing palliative care in the geriatric population, the author addresses 2 issues. First, it must be ascertained which medical conditions benefit from a palliative approach rather than more aggressive treatment, which is often called "life prolonging." Second, the focus must be on what patients and their families want. Even if a certain intervention may increase the chance of survival, the price of that intervention to quality of life may sway patients and families away from being aggressive.

Very few medical interventions in the elderly have a significant benefit, and many have substantial side effects. In many cases, there is not a distinct line between palliative care and life-extending care in the elderly regarding clinically significant outcomes. It is important to provide patients with accurate information about the risks and benefits of what their options are, and to support a more palliative approach if that is what they choose.

THE ELDERLY: DEMOGRAPHICS AND EXPECTATIONS

Who are the elderly? If Medicare criteria are used, people over the age of 65 qualify, and the number of those people is increasing, expected to constitute 20% of the population by 2050.[1] For the purposes of this article, though, the age of 75 will be used as a cutoff. There are many reasons for this distinction, primarily because there are

Disclosure: The author has nothing to disclose.
Personal Physician Care, 6334 Cedar Lane, Columbia, MD 21044, USA
E-mail address: alazris@ppcmd.com

Prim Care Clin Office Pract 46 (2019) 447–459
https://doi.org/10.1016/j.pop.2019.05.007
0095-4543/19/© 2019 Elsevier Inc. All rights reserved.

sparse data about health outcomes after this age. It is known that prognosis and the impact of intervention change at this age, as is clear in cancer screening. Similarly, the treatment of many chronic illnesses, such as diabetes and coronary artery disease, does not have good data to support aggressive treatment after age 75.

Because the vast amount of elderly die of and are disabled by chronic disease, that is where the focus should be when determining how to best care for them. Aggressive treatment of chronic illness leads a large number of elders to consume many medicines, see multiple specialists, and spend a significant amount of their last years in the hospital. There is evidence that aggressive treatment instigates deterioration in quality of life without necessarily prolonging life or ameliorating illness. The fact that almost half of the elderly spend time in the hospital during the last month of life is a testament to the fact that the expensive and aggressive care being touting is not effective.[2] More significantly, much of that care comes at a hefty price to the patient and health care dollars.

What do the elderly want? When asked, most suggest that the quality of their life is most important. Most want to die at home, not in the hospital.[3] Most do not want to be on so many medicines. Very often the pressures from family, from the medical system, or even from a lack of understanding of their options drive the elderly to pursue a more aggressive approach to care. Many elders also do not understand what palliative care is.[4] A large number associate it with end-of-life care and hospice. There is a natural assumption that those who take a palliative path are going to die more quickly than those who do not. If they understand the nature and effectiveness of palliation, many may pursue that route.

THE LIMITS OF AGGRESSIVE MEDICAL INTERVENTIONS IN THE ELDERLY

In their excellent book, *Medical Reversals*, Cifu and Prasad[5] make an important point that often is neglected by the medical community. Unless there is quality evidence that certain tests, procedures, or drugs help a specific population, then it should not be assumed that they do. In fact, it is often best to assume the opposite. Many standard treatments in younger people have not been demonstrated to be effective in the elderly, and few studies are done on patients older than 75 years old.[6] Also, elderly patients are a heterogenous group. Each is an individual with many chronic illnesses, symptoms, risks, and personal expectations. Even if a generic elderly population is studied, those results often do not help doctors care for the patient sitting in front of them.

A few examples are in order:

- Statin cholesterol medicines have been shown to prevent subsequent myocardial infarctions and cerebrovascular accidents in people with vascular disease or a high risk of having vascular disease.[7] However, does this also apply to the elderly? The answer is that despite some subgroup analysis, it is not known. It is known that statins can cause leg weakness, pain, and possibly falls, side effects particularly of concern to frail elders.[8]
- Although it was front-page news that ideal systolic blood pressure in the elderly should be pushed to less than 130, the data for such assumptions are moot. A single study found lower blood pressure to be efficacious in a younger group of elders who have very specific criteria,[9] whereas other studies in different populations found lower pressures to cause more death.[10] It is known that aggressive blood pressure control can cause dangerous hypotension, renal disease, falls, weakness, and worsening memory, among other issues related to the medicines themselves.[11]

- Although it is standard of care to give anticoagulation to avert strokes, the reality of that intervention is hazier. In fact, most studies do not even consider the impact of anticoagulation in people over the age of 80. Of the studies available, anticoagulation confers a benefit of preventing approximately 6 disabling strokes a year among 1000 people who use it, whereas 6 out of 1000 who use anticoagulation die or bleed in their brain and another 40 out of 1000 are hospitalized for major bleeds[12] (**Fig. 1**). In people prone to falling or bleeding, or in people who simply do not want to take a medicine with so little benefit, anticoagulation may not be appropriate, even if the patient wants to be aggressive in his or her care.

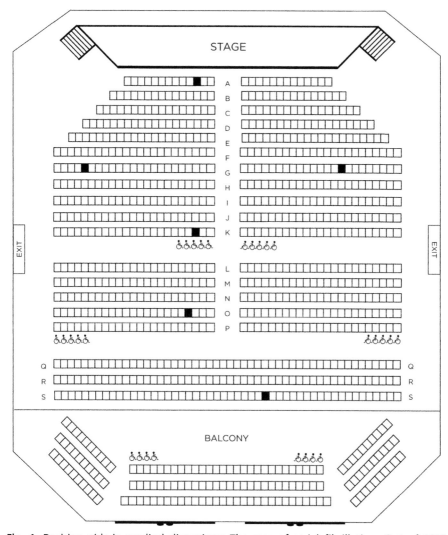

Fig. 1. Decision aids in medical discussions: The case of atrial fibrillation. Out of 1000 moderate-risk people in atrial fibrillation treated with anticoagulation compared with 1000 treated with aspirin, 6 will avoid a disabling stroke in a year, and 6 will either die or bleed in their brains.

Out of 1000 moderate-risk people in atrial fibrillation treated with anticoagulation compared with 1000 treated with aspirin, 6 will avoid a disabling stroke in a year, and 6 will either die or bleed in their brains.

A final caveat must be added regarding frailty. As people become burdened by their chronic medical conditions, many decline physically and mentally. Frailty is a physiologic condition characterized by debilitating symptoms in the absence of any specific cause of those changes (**Box 1**). It is estimated that more than 35% of people at least 85 years old suffer from frailty.[13] It is also known that the frailer an elder is, the worse will be his or her outcome, and the less likely aggressive medical interventions will be of value. Because chronic disease and aging take a toll on human bodies as the number of years a person has left to live diminishes, then aggressive care will have diminishing returns in terms of life-saving potential, while having an increasing propensity to cause harm. That is why a palliative approach is often the most medially prudent path to take, not one that compromises longevity for quality, but rather one that improves both.

WHAT IS GERIATRIC PALLIATIVE CARE?

According to the *Geriatric Palliative Care* textbook, palliative care for the elderly "focuses on providing patients with relief from the symptoms, pain, and stress of a serious illness, whatever the diagnosis may be. The goal is to improve quality of life for both the patient and family."[14] In other words, we want our patients to feel better and be more functional rather than attempting to "fix" their diseases. Too often in the medical culture, we are all about measuring and fixing numbers rather than providing compassionate care. Dennis McCullough's book,[15] *My Mother, Your Mother*, uses a different term to describe palliation: "slow medicine." He argues that aggressive medical care in the elderly is often counterproductive, especially in those with many chronic illnesses and frailty. Rather, one should treat the elderly slowly and cautiously, focusing more on symptom management and a gentle approach to care.

As Olser said: "Listen to the patient; he is telling you the diagnosis." We do not know what the ideal numbers should be in each elderly patient we treat, nor do we know what medicines, tests, and procedures may help the patient in front of us. Very often fixing 1 problem (lowering the blood pressure, treating cholesterol) can exacerbate another (worsening renal disease, increased leg pain/weakness). Therefore, we must rely on what the patient tells us and what we can observe. In effect, this is palliative care.

HOSPITALIZATION IN GERIATRIC PALLIATIVE CARE

Hospitalization is an area in which a palliative approach may make the most sense. Although certainly in the case of a broken hip or infected appendix, aggressive care

---

Box 1
Symptoms of frailty

Muscle weakness

Fatigue

Weight loss

Slow performance

Low activity

Cognitive decline

in the hospital may be lifesaving, many cases of hospitalization do not serve so clear a purpose and in fact may cause more harm than good. As mentioned, almost 40% of elders die in the hospital,[16] receiving expensive and ineffective care for diseases that may be served by a gentler approach. To put an elderly patient in the hospital because of common occurrences like syncope exposes that person to medication errors, infection, and overly aggressive care by a squadron of doctors who typically do not know the patient, without any proven benefit.[17,18] If a patient has dementia, the hospital itself accelerates memory loss and functional decline and increases the risk of delirium.[19–21] If a patient is frail, hospitalization similarly can be dangerous; fast medicine, as Dennis McCullough labels it, can throw a well-compensated frail elder into a state of rapid decline. There are very few chronic conditions in which hospitalization has been proven to be more beneficial than being treated at home among elders.[22] In almost all cases, potential dangers outweigh risks, showing again how a palliative approach is often the most sensible path to take.

A good example is congestive heart failure (CHF). It is known that outcomes in elders with CHF who are hospitalized and who have aggressive care are abysmal, with almost half not alive in a year.[23] In hospitals, elders often are overdiuresed, have urinary catheters and intravenous lines, and are subjected to infections, delirium, and medical errors. A study of elders with CHF who are kept at home and treated with a palliative approach shows that, when compared with those treated in an aggressive way, they have fewer exacerbations and less discomfort, and they live longer.[16]

THE ROLE OF THE PRIMARY CARE PHYSICIAN IN GERIATRIC PALLIATIVE CARE

Initiating palliative care is a role often best served by a patient's primary care physician. A patient's doctor can best explain the risks and benefits of medical interventions in light of their understanding of their patient's unique medical conditions. The primary care physician can help the patient design a path forward that is both medically sensible and palliative in scope. Often, the two go hand in hand. A simple approach to a palliative care discussion includes the following:

- Elucidating the patient's goals and objectives in the medical records
- Creating and updating advanced directives and power of attorney
- In the case of patients with dementia, involving families early in the discussion
- Clearly and accurately describing the risks and benefits of an aggressive approach versus a palliative approach for each of their chronic problems. This should include discussing the benefits and risks of specialists, of hospitalization, and of using medicines/tests/procedures to monitor and treat their chronic conditions. In all cases, assuring care coordination among different doctors and providers is important
- Discussing alternative approaches to aggressive care
- Discussing issues of safety, fall risk, ability to self-medicate, and depression
- Caregiver support when necessary

Very often a palliative approach can coexist with a more aggressive approach; a patient may have different expectations for various conditions. It is important that patients understand the implications of their various decisions, and that their goals and expectations be updated regularly as their condition changes. It is also crucial in a geriatric setting to involve caregivers without infringing on a patient's own decision-making capacity until that patient is deemed to lack capacity. Ultimately, if a patient has set goals and objectives and comprehends the implications of their decisions, then a physician's role is to assure compliance with the patient's plan of care.

DEMENTIA AS AN EXAMPLE OF A PALLIATIVE APPROACH

The diagnosis and treatment of dementia are illustrative of how the palliative approach to disease management works and how the lines between aggressive care and palliative care are often blurred. Dementia is one of the most rapidly growing diseases of the elderly,[24] and it is devastating to patients and caregivers. There are several classes of dementia[25] (**Table 1**), and each is treated somewhat uniquely. However, in fact, dementia has unique manifestations in each person, and an individualized approach often makes the most sense, despite what type of dementia the patient is stated to have.

What would be an aggressive approach to dementia? Typically, those with dementia will have a series of evaluations, including laboratory tests and computed tomographic/MRI scans, and will often follow with a neurologist. They will take "disease-altering" medicines, such as Donepezil (Aricept) or Memantine (Namenda), or the more recent combination of both, based on the stage of dementia (**Table 2**). How effective is this approach? The workup of dementia typically is not helpful; 6 cases of reversible dementia are found out of 1000 people tested, [26] and most of the few revealing tests are ordered by a patient's primary care doctor. The efficacy of disease-altering medications is suspect. Studies show a tiny divergence from placebo with these medicines when formal testing is done, and no difference from placebo when caregiver scores are considered. All studies on these medications end in a year, at which time placebo and pharmaceutical treatment are identical.[27]

How does a palliative approach differ? After basic laboratory tests and imaging studies to rule out reversible causes are performed, the essential objective is to help a patient's function and memory with the goal of prolonging independence and maintaining safety and dignity. A pharmaceutical-based and specialist-centered approach should be eschewed; dementia medicines, in addition to being ineffective, do have potential side effects. A recent study points to several interventions that do impact memory and function: stress reduction, Mediterranean diet, physical exercise, and good sleep.[28] A palliative approach will advocate these approaches, while focusing on patient comfort, safety, and behavior. The provider may work on memory techniques (writing everything down), socialization, and tending to the needs of caregivers.

The Functional Assessment Staging (FAST) scale[29] (**Box 2**), among others, can help physicians to ascertain when a patient with dementia will benefit from hospice. This ascertainment is not always easy; dementia is slowly debilitating, and patients may live many years. By using FAST criteria with other clinical parameters (**Table 3**), 62% of patients are correctly identified and survive less than 6 months.

Table 1 Classes of dementia	
Alzheimer disease (85% of dementias)	Slow onset, gradual but steady decline, no physical manifestations
Vascular (multi-infarct)	Variable onset, periods of rapid decline and then no decline, physical manifestation of stroke
Lewy body	Slow onset, fluctuating cognition, visual hallucinations, tremors, poor gait
Frontotemporal (Pick)	Younger onset, rapid progression, disinhibition, language problems, memory intact

Table 2 Stages of dementia	
Mild, early stage	Forgetfulness easily hidden, no cognitive deficits, could be normal memory loss of aging
Moderate	Memory loss more common and not concealed, personality changes, needs reminders and help
Severe	Very forgetful, dependent on caregivers for activities of daily living (ADLs), speech issues, some physical issues

PARKINSON DISEASE AS AN EXAMPLE OF A PALLIATIVE APPROACH

Parkinson disease is a progressive neurologic condition that leads to debility (**Table 4**). Pharmaceutical treatment of Parkinson can help to improve symptoms, but nothing available slows or prevents the progression of the disease.[30] Therefore, palliating symptoms, medicine side effects, and dangers from Parkinson is most crucial. Patients and their families should discuss with their primary care doctor likely disease progression, develop advanced directives especially regarding feeding tubes and artificial fluids, and regularly review safety issues, fall risk, functional decline, and mental status changes that may occur. It has been shown that frequent physical therapy can help preserve function and reduce fall risk; both occupational and speech therapy can address common symptoms of Parkinson.[31,32] Also, given the very high prevalence of depression, memory loss, bladder dysfunction, and pain in Parkinson patients, these physical manifestations of disease should be addressed in a palliative way.

ARTHRITIS AS AN EXAMPLE OF A PALLIATIVE APPROACH

Arthritis is a leading cause of disability and pain in the elderly.[14] Consistent with palliation in the elderly in general, treatment of arthritis does not typically require specialty visits, radiographs, or hospitalization; rather it focuses on alleviation of pain and improvement in function. Physical therapy and exercise help achieve both goals, especially when coupled with occupational therapy and home evaluation.[33,34] If pharmaceuticals are used, these will need to be introduced judiciously, with risks and benefits assessed and discussed for each medicine considered. Assistive devices and fall-prevention strategies should be part of any arthritis program. Ultimately, rather than testing and looking for cause, a palliative approach for arthritis involves an individualized comprehensive program to address symptoms and their ramifications. Specialty consultation is most useful if joint injections and surgery are being considered.

Box 2 Functional assessment staging scale 1 to 6

1. No difficulty objectively or subjectively

2. Forgetting location of items, subjective work problems

3. Noticeable decline in job function, difficulty traveling to new locations

4. Decreased ability in performance of complex tasks

5. Requires assistance in choosing appropriate clothing

6. Occasionally or regularly improperly putting on clothing, bathing properly, toileting correctly; having urinary or fecal incontinence

Table 3 Functional assessment staging 7 and hospice criteria for dementia: 1 functional assessment staging scale 7 symptom (on left) plus 1 item (on right)	
A: Speech limited to 6 or fewer words	Severe infection, such as sepsis or pyelonephritis
B: Speech limited to 1 word	Aspiration pneumonia
C: Unable to ambulate without assistance	Multiple pressure ulcers
D: Unable to sit up without assistance	10% weight loss or albumin <2.5
E: Unable to smile	
F: Unable to hold up head independently	

PNEUMONIA AND ASPIRATION AS AN EXAMPLE OF A PALLIATIVE APPROACH

Pneumonia is one of the most common causes of hospitalization and death in the elderly. An aggressive approach to care involves imaging, specialty consultation, and hospitalization usually with intravenous antibiotics. A study of elderly patients with frailty showed that a palliative approach to pneumonia, including home treatment, afforded better outcomes with more preserved function than did hospitalization.[35–37] Home-treated patients die less, have less delirium, and recover more quickly. Home oxygen, home health care, antibiotics, and relief of symptoms can all be accomplished in a home environment; hospitalization introduces substantial risk without proven benefit to frail and confused elders.

Aspiration pneumonia is common in patients with dementia, strokes, high levels of frailty, and various neuromuscular conditions. Speech therapy and dietary modification can help prevent aspiration in patients prone to it. The use of tube feeding in these patients does not improve outcome and leads to both discomfort and adverse events, and it should be avoided.[38] Often patients (or their families) seek to eat liberally despite the risk of aspiration; in such situations, comfort feeding can help people feel better, and symptoms can be controlled with medications, nebulizers, and oxygen.

UNIVERSAL PRINCIPLES OF GERIATRIC PALLIATIVE CARE

A truism of geriatric care is that less is better. Fewer medications, tests, consultants, procedures, and hospitalizations often translate to a better quality and quantity of life. It is known from Medicare data that elderly who have less access to specialty care and more primary care are likely to live longer and better.[39–41] Palliative primary care

Table 4 Stages of Parkinson disease	
1. Unilateral tremor or movement disorder, changes in posture	Remains independent in ADLs
2. Bilateral tremor or movement disorder, rigidity, ataxia	Can live alone, some ADL impairment
3. Worse gait, high fall risk, slow moving	Independent with some home aides, occupational therapy
4. Limiting symptoms, needs assistive device to walk, hard to move	Needs physical help to live alone
5. Difficult to stand/walk, needs wheelchair, delusions, swallowing problems	Needs round-the-clock assistance

stresses shared decision making and an individualized patient-centric approach. A few concrete examples are as follows:

1. *Reduction of polypharmacy:* For every disease and symptom, there are multiple medications and supplements that are alleged to be either necessary or helpful. Many medications in the elderly have a marginal benefit, as was shown in the case of anticoagulation and statins. As William Osler says: "If you have a problem and you treat it with a medicine, now you have 2 problems." Still, because of the number of chronic diseases that inflict the elderly, and the number of specialists many of them see, elders typically are on large numbers of medicines/supplements. The average elder is on 12 medicines. When medicines are combined in an aged body, side effects are accentuated; studies show that the more medicines older people take, the more likely they are to suffer from weakness, falls, worse mentation, and depression among others.[42,43] Thus, a basic rule of palliative care is to use medicines that help people feel better and have increased function, but to avoid excessive medicines that are given to allegedly prolong life. Certainly, there are medicines one may use that do not adhere to those rules explicitly, such as medicines for blood pressure. However, if antihypertensives cause patients to feel worse, then a palliative approach would favor a higher pressure if that results in improved symptoms. Discussing the actual benefits and risks of pharmaceutical treatment with patients helps to shorten medication lists and improve patient well-being without necessarily impacting survival. Deprescribing medicines can be difficult and requires an accurate discussion of risks/benefits, consultation with specialists, and review of possible consequences of medication withdrawal[44] (**Table 5**).

2. *Fall prevention:* There is nothing more painful and more likely to cause functional decline in the elderly than falls. Falls are the fifth leading cause of death in the elderly and one of the top causes of disability and decline.[14] Any palliative approach to care must be cognizant of the need to prevent falls. The role of excessive medications in falls is of paramount concern.[45] When discussing risks and benefits of medicines, a provider needs to address the increased fall risk of medications and their combination. For instance, being on an anxiety medicine, a blood pressure medicine, and a statin all can increase the chance of falling, so a palliative discussion may lead to the reduction or removal of one or more of these medications if the patient has poor gait or poor judgment. In addition, a positive approach to fall reduction is crucial. Assessing a history of falls, the situation of a patient's home (clutter, throw rugs), and the need for an assistive device should all be done on a regular basis, often at the annual wellness visit, and more frequently if

Table 5 Strategies for deprescribing	
Review the actual benefit of the medication	Use decision aids to show true benefits, individualized for patient's age and comorbidity
Review the potential risks of the medication	Discuss how the medication can cause harm and side effects, personalize it to the patient's condition
Review medicine interactions	This should be done with supplements as well
Work with specialist providers	Often specialists are less likely to deprescribe, and patients are reassured if they are involved
Discuss possible ramifications of deprescribing	Both real and placebo effects can occur when medications are stopped, discuss in advance

the patient has a fall. The use of grab bars, home health assessments, physical therapy, and exercise programs can also help to avert falls.

3. *Recognizing depression*: Both depression and anxiety are common conditions of the elderly, the prevalence being 5% to 10% and substantially higher in those who have chronic illness and frailty.[46] The aggressive and palliative approaches to these conditions are similar: the goal is to use medicines and psychological interventions to mitigate symptoms and help people to feel better. The symptoms of depression (fatigue, weakness, lack of interest, weight loss, sleep disorder) mimic those of frailty and chronic disease, so often it is difficult to distinguish one from another. Treating for depression with pharmaceuticals and psychotherapy has been shown to be effective in the elderly.[14] Often psychotherapy is not appropriate for those with dementia or other issues of memory loss, whereas medications have serious side effects that can impact mentation, fall risk, energy level, sleep, eating/weight, and organ function. An individualized approach to depression and anxiety is crucial; some elders do best with very low-dose medicines, whereas others need extremely high doses. Many elderly people have sleep disorders with or without depression; the prevalence can be as high as 50% to 70%.[47] Often this needs to be addressed independently of depression, focusing on sleep hygiene and cognitive behavior therapy.

4. *Achieving maximal functional status*: Surveys of elders consistently find that they are happiest if they stay at home.[48] To do this, they will need to be able to function independently or with some degree of assistance. A full assessment of their activities of daily living and independent assessment of daily living is a good way to start. When deficiencies are revealed, a plan can be put in place to help ameliorate them. For instance, if a patient has a difficult time getting dressed, then an occupational therapist can assess the home situation, providing solutions. In most cases, an exercise program and fall reduction plan are necessary to help people achieve maximal functional status. From a more social perspective, knowing how patients are able to buy and cook food, get to doctor appointments, buy/afford medicines, and carry out basic daily activities are important to assess at least once a year. Often for such discussions, caregivers should be involved.

5. *Reduction of discomfort*: The alleviation of pain is a paramount concern in any palliative approach. This could be physical or emotional discomfort. The author addresses some of these issues in discussing arthritis. Ultimately, pain is a salient barrier to function, memory, comfort, and quality of life. A few basic principles are as follows:
   - Searching for an underlying cause of discomfort is only important if finding and fixing that cause helps to alleviate the discomfort, and if the patient/family would want to pursue that approach.
   - Medicines for discomfort need to be assessed for their risks and benefits before being used, and generally the use of medicines with many side effects should be the last resort, especially if they cause falls, confusion, or loss of function. In fact, the reduction of medications can help to alleviate discomfort.
   - Often changes in environment, physical activity, socialization, and stress reduction can help with pain and mental anguish. Pain can be a manifestation of anxiety.

6. *Do not be aggressive*: When we are treating someone palliatively, we do not focus on tests and number measurements. Stressing tight control of sugar or blood pressure, measuring cholesterol and ordering multiple laboratory tests, and screening for cancer or carotid/heart disease in the absence of symptoms are counterproductive to a palliative approach. Excessive testing and measuring can lead to

stress and does not alleviate discomfort; there is little evidence this approach leads to life prolongation or the prevention of disease in the elderly. Similarly, as discussed, hospitalization often causes more distress and poorer outcomes than keeping a patient at home. Ultimately, medicines, tests, procedures, and hospital visits should be considered if they can help a patient feel better, function at a higher level, and avoid a deterioration of a chronic disease that may lead to disability or discomfort.

SUMMARY

In the elderly, there is scant evidence that aggressive medical care is always more effective that a palliative approach. Medicines, hospitalization, and other interventions should be discussed before prescribed. Palliative care addresses many of the issues that are most important for elders to remain comfortable, retain their functional capacity, and stay independent.

REFERENCES

1. Strestha LB, Heisler EJ. The changing demographic profile of the United States. Washington, DC: Congressional Research Service; 2011. p. 13–8.
2. Jennings B. Health care costs in end of life and palliative care: the quest for ethical reform. J Soc Work 2011;7:300–17.
3. Byock I. The best care possible. New York: Avery; 2012. p. 3.
4. Hoerger M, Perry LM, Gramling R, et al. Does educating patients about the early palliative care study increase preferences for outpatient palliative cancer care? findings from project EMPOWER. Health Psychol 2017;36(6):538–48.
5. Cifu A, Prasad V. Ending medical reversals: improving outcomes, saving lives. Baltimore (MD): Johns Hopkins University Press; 2015. 149, 150, 193.
6. Hadler N. Rethinking aging. Chapel Hill (NC): University of North Carolina Press; 2011. p. 190.
7. Collins R, Reith C, Emberson J, et al. Interpretation of the evidence for the efficacy and safety of statin therapy. Lancet 2016;388:2532–61.
8. Odden MC, Pletcher MJ, Coxson PG, et al. Cost-effectiveness and population impact of statins for primary prevention in adults aged 75 years or older in the United States. Ann Intern Med 2015;162(8):533–41.
9. The Sprint Research Group. A randomized trial of intensive versus standard blood-pressure control. N Engl J Med 2015;373:2103–16.
10. Chrysant SG. Aggressive systolic blood pressure control in older subjects: benefits and risks. Postgrad Med 2018;130(2):159–65.
11. Lazris A. Curing medicare. Ithaca (NY): Cornell University Press; 2016. p. 28–32.
12. Rifkin E, Lazris A. Interpreting health benefits and risks. New York, New York: Springer Press; 2015. p. 95–104.
13. Chai E, Meier D, Morris J, et al. Geriatric palliative care. New York: Oxford University Press; 2014. p. 317.
14. Chai E, Meier D, Morris J, et al. Geriatric palliative care. New York: Oxford University Press; 2014. p. 3–9, 461–66, 321, 328.
15. McCullough D. My mother, your mother. New York: Harper Books; 2012.
16. Byock. The best care possible. New York: Avery; 2012. p. 107–9.
17. Brownlee S. Overtreated: why too much medicine is making us sicker and poorer. New York: Bloomsbury Press; 2007. p. 47, 52.
18. Bernstein L. 1 in 25 Hospital patients gets an infection during treatment, CDC Reports 2014. p. A3. Washington Post.

19. Ehlenbach WJ. Association between acute care and critical illness hospitalization and cognitive function in older adults. JAMA 2010;303(8):763–7.
20. Witlox J. Delirium in elderly patients and the risk of post discharge mortality. JAMA 2010;304(4):443–51.
21. Pedone C. Elderly patients with cognitive impairment have a high risk for functional decline during hospitalization. J Gerontol A Biol Sci Med Sci 2005;12:1576–80.
22. Lazris. Curing medicare. Ithaca (NY): Cornell University Press; 2016. p. 110–21.
23. Curtis LH. Early and long-term outcomes of heart failure in elderly persons, 2001-2005. Arch Intern Med 2008;168(22):2481–5.
24. Available at: https://www.alz.org/alzheimers-dementia/facts-figures; http://act.alz.org/site/DocServer/112114_Most_Expensive_Disease_Handout.pdf?docID=40161. Accessed February 1, 2019.
25. Available at: https://www.nia.nih.gov/health/types-dementia 2219-29. Accessed February 1, 2019.
26. Mark-Clarfield A. The decreasing prevalence of reversible dementias an updated meta-analysis. Arch Intern Med 2003;163(18):2219–29.
27. Rifkin E, Lazris A. Interpreting health benefits and risks. (New York, New York): Springer Press; 2015. p. 161–71.
28. Bredesen DE, Amos EC, Canick J, et al. Reversal of cognitive decline in Alzheimer's disease. Aging 2016;8(6):1250–8.
29. Available at: https://www.mccare.com/pdf/fast.pdf. Accessed February 1, 2019.
30. Available at: http://www.parkinson.org/Understanding-Parkinsons/What-is-Parkinsons/Stages-of-Parkinsons. Accessed February 1, 2019.
31. De Goede CJ. The effects of physical therapy in Parkinson's disease: a research synthesis. Arch Phys Med Rehabil 2001;82(4):509–15.
32. Borrione P. Effects of physical activity in Parkinson's disease: a new tool for rehabilitation. World J Methodol 2014;4(3):133–43.
33. Minor MA. Exercise in the treatment of osteoarthritis. Rheum Dis Clin North Am 1999;25(2):397–415.
34. Ettinger WHJ, Burns R, Messier SP, et al. "A randomized trial comparing aerobic exercise and resistance exercise with a health education program in older adults with knee osteoarthritis" The Fitness Arthritis and Seniors Trial (FAST). JAMA 1991;277(1):25–31.
35. Kruse RL. Does hospitalization impact survival after lower respiratory infection in nursing home residents? Med Care 2004;42:860–70.
36. Loeb M. Effect of a clinical pathway to reduce hospitalization in nursing home residents with pneumonia. JAMA 2006;295(21):2503–10.
37. Givens JL. Survival and comfort after treatment of pneumonia in advanced dementia. Arch Intern Med 2011;171(3):217.
38. Finucane T, Bynum J. Use of tube feeding to prevent aspiration pneumonia. Lancet 1996;348:1421–4.
39. Macinko J, Starfield B, Shi L. Quantifying the health benefit of primary care physician supply in the United States. Int J Health Serv 2007;37(1):111–26.
40. Wennberg JE. Executive summary of tracking the care of patients with severe chronic illnesses: the Dartmouth atlas of health care. Hanover (Germany): Dartmouth Institute for Policy and clinical Practice, Center for Health Policy Research; 2008.
41. Wennberg JE, Fischer ES, Skinner JS. "Geography and the debate over medicare reform," Health Affairs 2002. p. 96–114.
42. Gurwitz JH. Incidence and preventability of adverse drug events among older persons. JAMA 2003;289(9):1107–16.

43. Routledge P. Adverse drug reactions in elderly patients. Br J Clin Pharmacol 2004;57(2):121–6.
44. Scott IA, Hilmer SN, Reeve E, et al. Reducing inappropriate polypharmacy: the process of deprescribing. JAMA Intern Med 2015;175(5):827–34.
45. Lipsitz L. Causes and correlates of recurrent falls in ambulatory frail elderly. J Gerontol 1991;46(4):114–22.
46. Periyakoil VJ, Hallenback J. Identifying and managing preparatory grief and depression in end of life. Am Fam Physician 2002;65:883–90.
47. Hugel H, Ellershaw JE, Cook L, et al. The prevalence, key causes, and management of insomnia in palliative care patients. J Pain Symptom Manage 2004;27(4): 316–21.
48. Mhaske R. Happiness and aging. J Psychosoc Res 2017;12(1):71–9.

Pediatric Palliative Care

Sarah Norris, MD, MEd[a],*, Sheera Minkowitz, MD, MBA[b],
Kathryn Scharbach, MD, MS[c]

KEYWORDS

- Pediatric palliative care • Total pain • Nonpharmacologic therapies • End-of-life care
- Bereavement

KEY POINTS

- The field of pediatric palliative and hospice medicine describes a care approach that aims to relieve total pain and improve quality of life of both children and their families through team based care.
- Introduction of pediatric palliative care is appropriate and optimal at the time a serious condition presents.
- Total pain encompasses physical, emotional, social, and spiritual pain.
- Medical management of pediatric patients focuses on appropriate pain and symptom using tools validated in the pediatric population and specific pediatric-based dosing.
- Excellent communication that promotes patient-centered and family-centered shared decision-making is paramount when establishing goals of care and may include acute goals in addition to end-of-life discussions.

INTRODUCTION

Pediatric hospice and palliative medicine is a field of medical expertise that aims to relieve total pain and improve the quality of life of children and families. Shared decision-making and care coordination for children and their families living with a serious illness is a hallmark of the field. Regardless of prognosis, the introduction of palliative care is appropriate, and often optimal, at the moment a serious condition presents. Pediatric palliative care team members often include medical providers, social workers, chaplains, child life specialists, music therapists, art therapists, and psychologists. The interdisciplinary team approach aspires to address the full range of needs experienced by patients and families across inpatient, outpatient, and home settings.[1]

Disclosure Statement: The authors have nothing to disclose.
[a] Children's Hospital at Montefiore, 3415 Bainbridge Avenue, Bronx, NY 10467, USA; [b] Division of Pediatric Hematology/Oncology, The Children's Hospital at Montefiore, 3411 Wayne Avenue, Bronx, NY 10467, USA; [c] Icahn School of Medicine at Mount Sinai, One Gustave Levy Place Box 1202a, New York, NY 10029, USA
* Corresponding author.
E-mail address: sanorri@montefiore.org

TOTAL PAIN: PHYSICAL, SOCIAL, EMOTIONAL, AND SPIRITUAL ASPECTS OF PAIN

Patients are more than a medical condition. Entering the medical world often diminishes the individual to their presentation or diagnosis. Palliative care preserves the personhood by recognizing total pain and aggressively treating it. When parents and caregivers have been asked to share their goals for the hospitalization of their child, treatment of pain was second only to accurate diagnosis.[2]

The experience of physical pain is modified by the social context, emotional impact, and meaning assigned to pain. Broadening the assessment to account for these influences (**Fig. 1**) allows for creation of a multimodal treatment plan that encompasses

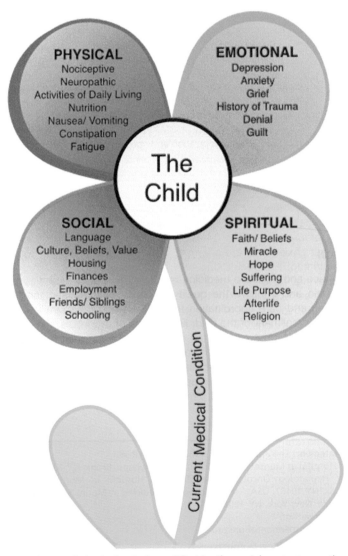

PHYSICAL
Nociceptive
Neuropathic
Activities of Daily Living
Nutrition
Nausea/ Vomiting
Constipation
Fatigue

EMOTIONAL
Depression
Anxiety
Grief
History of Trauma
Denial
Guilt

The Child

SOCIAL
Language
Culture, Beliefs, Value
Housing
Finances
Employment
Friends/ Siblings
Schooling

SPIRITUAL
Faith/ Beliefs
Miracle
Hope
Suffering
Life Purpose
Afterlife
Religion

Current Medical Condition

Fig. 1. The experience of physical pain is modified by the social context, emotional impact, and meaning assigned to pain.

pharmacologic and nonpharmacologic interventions. Comprehensive total pain assessment enables palliative care teams to partner with the primary team to ground goals of care.

PHYSICAL PAIN

Physical pain is nociceptive or neuropathic. Nociceptive pain indicates tissue injury or inflammation and is often described as dull or throbbing. It is frequently improved with nonsteroidal anti-inflammatory medications (NSAIDs) and opioids. Neuropathic pain (centrally or peripherally mediated) reflects abnormal excitability and is frequently described as electric, sharp, or shooting. It can persist long after an injury and can be very difficult to treat. Neuropathic pain is often poorly responsive to opioids and NSAIDs. Often a child with neuropathic pain responds better to integrative therapies, including physical therapy, to promote continued mobility and cognitive behavioral therapies (visualization and body scanning) to promote self-modulation of pain and sense of body control. Pharmacologic agents, such as anticonvulsants (gabapentin), tricyclic antidepressants (amitriptyline), and serotonin-norepinephrine reuptake inhibitors (SNRIs) (duloxetine) should be viewed as adjuvants in a multimodal pain plan.

The gold standard for pain assessment is self-report. Not all children are verbal, so input from the primary caregiver is crucial in understanding a child's pain manifestations. Chronic pain in children is often not accompanied by vital sign changes or behavioral changes commonly associated with pain (withdrawing from the environment or crying), as they have learned to sleep or play despite pain.

Age-Related Considerations

Young infants may show pain by crying, stiffening their bodies, withdrawing to painful stimuli, or with facial grimace (brow bulge, eyes squeezed shut, mouth open, exaggerated nasolabial furrow). Toward the latter half of their first year, infants will begin to exhibit stranger anxiety and are often best assessed while in their caregiver's arms. The Neonatal/Infant Pain Scale can be used in children younger than 1 year old. Similar to older infants, toddlers (age 1–3 years) can exhibit significant stranger anxiety and are often best evaluated initially by simple observation while they roam within a safe space equipped with developmentally appropriate props (eg, toys, colorful pictures, puppets). If the child is verbal, first identify what terms are used for pain in the child's home before questioning the child directly. The FLACC (Face, Legs, Activity, Cry, Consolability) can be used in children 2 months to 7 years of age.

Preschoolers (3–6 years) also may exhibit stranger anxiety. They can be reasonable self-reporters of pain if they are verbal and trust the provider. Occasionally at this age, children may be uncooperative with self-reporting and the clinician must fall back to observation, caregiver reports, and scales for nonverbal children (FLACC or revised FLACC [R-FLACC]). The R-FLACC is used for children with cognitive impairment. The FACES pain rating scale is a self-report scale for use in children 3 years and older. It includes 6 faces that start with a happy face and progresses to a crying face. Clinicians explain to the child that the first face has no pain, the second face has a little pain, the third face has a little more pain, the fourth has more pain still, the fifth face has a lot of pain, and the sixth face is the worst pain ever, but the child need not be crying to experience the worst pain ever. Then the child is asked which face best describes how he or she feels. The faces are anchored with even numbers from 0 to 10 for a numerical score. Because sometimes FACES can be assigned the numbers 0 to 5,[3] it is important to document the numerical score and the scale range (ie, 3 of 5). Similarly, the Oucher scale uses real photographs of children's faces and is available in gender-specific and racial/ethnic-specific versions.[4] School-age children 7 years and older can generally use a 0 to 10 numerical pain scale, visual analog scale, or verbal report scale similar to those used in adults.

Children with severe neurologic impairment frequently have underrecognized and thus undertreated pain. Parents of children with progressive metabolic, genetic, or noncurable neurologic conditions often report that their children experience symptoms of pain, feeding problems, and sleep problems. Chronic pain can impact all aspects of life and reinforce a cycle of fatigue, sleep disturbances, and family stress. Assessment tools like the R-FLACC allow for families to customize the tool to reflect their child's pain behaviors. It is important to examine children without clothing on at each visit to identify any cause of pain/discomfort. Diagnostic tests may be useful in children with verbal communication challenges and may guide the team toward identifiable, treatable sources of pain[5]

Principles of Physical Pain Management

The World Health Organization recommends a 2-step approach for treating pain. Step 1 for mild pain: provide adjuvants (like hot/cold packs, repositioning) and acetaminophen or nonsteroidal agents. Step 2 for moderate to severe pain: consider the addition of an opioid. Consider the principles in when prescribing medications.

Many young children or those with dysphagia are unable to swallow pills **Box 1**, so liquid and rectal formulations must be used. Liquid oral morphine is a good option for children with significant pain that would benefit from dosing that is more flexible than that offered by tablets. The only long-acting oral liquid opioid available in the United States is methadone. Extended-release morphine capsules are available that can be opened and sprinkled into food, but if accidently chewed, there is a risk of lethal overdose. Taste is also a consideration when prescribing medication to children, as some will refuse if they dislike the taste. Masking aversive tasting medication can be accomplished in chocolate or strawberry syrup. Pills that can be crushed can be stirred into pudding or other soft foods. Rarely, a nasogastric tube is necessary to assist with medication delivery, particularly if the medication is vital to the child's care and it is viewed as the least noxious method of obtaining the medication from the point of view of the child. Some children, especially when ill with mucositis or nausea, cannot tolerate oral medication. In these instances, transdermal or intravenous routes need to be considered. Rectal, subcutaneous, and intramuscular routes of administration of pain medication are avoided in children when possible.

Opioid-induced side effects in children include allergic reactions, constipation, delirium/confusion/hallucinations, nausea/vomiting, pruritus, myoclonic jerking, respiratory depression, and sedation. True allergic reactions are rare and important to distinguish (difficulty breathing, rash, hives). Pruritus without allergic reaction is best treated with opioid antagonists, not antihistamines. Consider opioid rotation if severe pruritis occurs, as not all opioids induce the same degree of pruritus. Children with

---

Box 1
Pediatric tips for pain management

Codeine and tramadol are no longer recommended for children

Dosing should be weight-based up to 50 kg when adult dosing can be used

When body mass index is >30, consider ideal weight when dosing opioids

Integrate nonpharmacological interventions and techniques, such as distraction, into each plan

refractory pain may benefit from regional anesthetics, reversible blockades with local anesthetics, neuroleptic agents, or radiofrequency ablation.[6]

Nonpharmacologic Therapies

Nonpharmacologic therapies augment symptom management, especially in the treatment of pain and anxiety. They range from simple caregiver maneuvers, such as cuddling and providing general social support, to more technical interventions, such as acupuncture.[7] Teaching of cognitive behavior techniques, such as hypnosis, guided imagery, biofeedback, and mindfulness-based stress reduction, have demonstrated efficacy in the treatment of pain and stress.[8,9] Child life specialists who are trained to provide developmentally normative play and help children cope with medical stress can be essential. Yoga and massage have been shown to be effective for reducing anxiety and pain.[9,10] Art therapy and music therapy may improve general well-being in terminally ill patients.[11] Acupuncture has been shown to be helpful in the treatment of chemotherapy-induced nausea and vomiting, and in pain, in children.[11,12] In addition, heating pads, or sometimes cold packs, can also help to relieve pain.[7] Aromatherapy may help with nausea.[13] Improving sleep hygiene also can attenuate pain and anxiety symptoms.

Anorexia/Cachexia/Weight Loss

From the time a child is born, weight is used as a marker of wellness. In the setting of serious illness, children may not be allowed to eat by mouth, they may lose the physical ability to eat by mouth, or they may become disinterested in eating because of pain or depression. Weight loss is very common and frequently distressing for patients and families. Loss of appetite has been shown to occur in up to 80% of pediatric patients with terminal cancer and is common in pediatric patients with acquired immunodeficiency syndrome, cardiac disease, lung disease, and complex chronic conditions. When appetite stimulation is desired, a limited range of pharmacologic interventions exist: megestrol acetate, cannabinoids, cyproheptadine, mirtazapine, and steroids. Although they may stimulate appetite, they will not necessarily induce weight gain.

Dietary assessment should include exploration into family rituals around meals and cooking styles. Hospitalized children often refuse unfamiliar food and lack appropriate tools (adaptive utensils, sippy cups) typically used in the home. Create meal plans that reflect patient preferences. If a child is not able to eat by mouth, then feeding tubes, orogastric, nasogastric, gastrointestinal, and duodenal, may be used. In some settings, parenteral nutrition is used via a central catheter. The use of long-term feeding assistance is often a difficult decision for patients and families. Losing the ability to eat by mouth may highlight the seriousness of the illness. It is frequently helpful to discuss the concept of pleasure feeding in which a child takes limited amounts by mouth while receiving most of the calories/nutrients through a tube. For many, preserving the ability to taste food is vital and supports the social connection associated with meals.

Delirium

Children in the intensive care unit (ICU) can experience delirium. Those at highest risk are younger than 2 years, have a high severity of illness, are being mechanically ventilated, and have developmental delay. Precipitating environmental factors include medication/treatment-related (benzodiazepines, cardiac bypass surgery, prolonged ICU stay, immobilization, and use of restraints). The Cornell Assessment of Pediatric Delirium has been validated in children from birth to 21 years old independent of presence/absence of developmental delay. This is an observational tool that provides a longitudinal measure of interactions/behaviors/response over 8 to 12 hours. To effectively treat delirium, the root cause needs to be identified. Common triggers include infection, hypoxemia, poor pain control, and metabolic abnormalities. First-line measures for treatment/prevention include optimizing pain control, using sedatives sparingly, avoiding restraints, allowing for early mobilization, providing cognitive stimulation during the day, and supporting sleep at night. Supporting sleep hygiene includes sunlight exposure during the day, minimizing light and noise overnight, and clustering care to minimize wakening. Medications that may be considered for treatment of delirium include dexmedetomidine, clonidine, and atypical antipsychotics.[14] Early recognition of delirium will lead to improved outcomes and decreased overall morbidity.

EMOTIONAL PAIN

When serious or life-changing news is shared, fear, sadness, anger, confusion, and a sense of feeling overwhelmed are common. In the evaluation of a child and family, it is important to screen for anxiety, depression, prior trauma, substance use, and domestic violence. Through understanding the primary caregiver's and patient's emotional state, a more supportive plan can be developed for the family that can lessen the burden of serious illness.[15]

Chronically or terminally ill children present with various physical symptoms, which are difficult for the children, parents, and their treating physicians to discern as being related to depressive or anxiety symptoms versus to their medical illness or interventions.[16] Physical and emotional symptoms are interrelated, and each symptom must be addressed accordingly. There is strong evidence that physicians underestimate the symptoms of depression and anxiety in adolescent patients with cancer, as well as in other children with chronic illnesses.[17–19]

Children with depressive or anxious symptoms should be evaluated with the Patient Health Questionnaire for Depression, the Children's Depression Inventory, the Memorial Symptom Assessment Scale, or the UCLA Posttraumatic Stress Disorder Reaction Index.[20,21] Treatment is always multimodal and needs to involve therapy, such as art therapy and/or standard psychotherapy. If the patient requires pharmacologic support for depression, the Food and Drug Administration indicates fluoxetine and escitalopram for use in the treatment of adolescent depression. The reliance on antidepressants without therapy will likely lead to suboptimal results and hinder the return to premorbid functioning.[17] For a psychiatric disorder of anxiety, various cognitive-behavioral interventions are recommended, including cognitive restructuring, and increasing available coping resources through teaching relaxation, problem-solving, and stress management.[22] In the cases of both depression and anxiety, the use of psychotropic medications, such as selective serotonin reuptake inhibitors or SNRIs, must be done with the utmost caution and with close monitoring due to the increased risk of suicide, the possibility of bringing about manic episodes, impact on liver functioning, and other possible complications.[23] Medication effectiveness should be assessed every 2 to 4 weeks, always beginning at low doses and titrating to response. At each visit, suicidal ideation should be evaluated along with other common side effects: abdominal pain, sleep disturbance, and headaches. Management of psychiatric diagnosis along with life-threatening or life-limiting illnesses requires a multimodal approach that involves the care of the entire family system.

SPIRITUAL PAIN

Spirituality is essential to children and families coping with serious illness.[24] To understand patients'/families' perception of illnesses and treatment, the meaning they assign to the relationship between themselves and a greater power must be appreciated. Spirituality and religiosity are distinct entities. A religion is an organized group that agrees to general tenants, whereas the meaning found in the practice might be described as spirituality. Spirituality encompasses both how humans practice their faith and find meaning in life, pain and illness. Providers often feel helpless when families use words they perceive to be strictly religious, such as "God" or "miracle."

Most parents of children facing serious illness want to have spiritual needs assessed and do not find it offensive. Completion of this assessment results in a perceived sense of higher support from the care team.[25] Spiritual challenges that arise for parents include questioning the meaning of faith or trying to make sense of why; feeling anger or blame toward God; or moving away from or rejecting their faith.[26] Understanding a patient/family in the context of their spirituality will be immensely helpful in addressing an individual's experience of pain and suffering.

SOCIAL PAIN

The child's experience of pain and illness is informed by the society in which the child lives, which starts with the family or home in which the child lives. Establishing preferred language and personal pronouns at the start of an encounter is essential. The use of interpreter services is essential if the provider does not speak the preferred language of the patient. Gender identity is best asked directly by asking about preferred personal pronouns (eg, he/him, she/her, they/them) directly. A comprehensive social assessment allows for a more informed and effective plan for addressing total pain.

A frequently used social history tool, the adolescent Home & Environment, Education & Employment, Activities, Drugs, Sexuality, Suicide/Depression (HEADSS) assessment (https://brightfutures.aap.org/Bright%20Futures%20Documents/History, %20Observation,%20and%20Surveillance.pdf) can be used for an assessment of any patient and family. The newer HEADS AT tool[27] was designed for use with children with medical complexity.

GOALS OF CARE

Families enter the health care system at different points in the diagnostic and therapeutic continuum. This may be at a time of diagnostic uncertainty, such as fetal consults for suspected cardiac defects or inherited life-threatening illnesses. They may have received a diagnosis for which the prognosis is uncertain, as in the case of children who are awaiting solid organ transplants, many oncologic diagnoses, cardiac anomalies, and immunologic deficiencies, such as human immunodeficiency virus. They may have received a diagnosis that will lead to a shortened life, as is the case with short gut syndrome, degenerative neurologic syndromes, cancers for which treatment has been unsuccessful, and children dependent on advanced technologies (feeding tubes, mechanical ventilation, cardiac assist devices, and renal replacement therapies). The foundation for setting goals of care is establishing effective communication that promotes patient-centered and family-centered shared decision-making.

Family Perspective

When a patient and family first hear unexpected news, they frequently express feeling overwhelmed.[28] Families may have a grief reaction as they mourn what they dreamt of[29] and are confronted with the possible death of their child or the potential of lasting impairment. In a span of moments the dreams they have for their children are abruptly challenged.

Parents suggest the following for improving provider-family communication: address the patient using the patient's first name and treat the patient as an individual; provide consistent care teams; acknowledge the family's role on the team and elicit an understanding of medical literacy to demonstrate respect for the parents' knowledge of the child[1]; and avoid euphemisms, which promote misunderstanding. Parents value physicians who they perceive as available, accountable, open to being questioned, allowing for hope, and focusing attention on the suffering of the child.

Parents of seriously ill children frequently desire to be treated as partners in their children's care alongside the medical team. It is useful to begin the conversation using the question, "What do you need to do to be a good parent to your child?" Parents offer answers that include the following: helping their child to feel loved through physical presence; advocating for them with the medical team, which may mean being present at patient rounds; and making medically informed and unselfish decisions while ensuring their spiritual wellness.[30] Parental responses provide insight to the care team on how their recommendations may impact parents' expressed duties as parents.

Families often face anxiety and denial, whereas providers are often anxious and feel ill-equipped to deal with the strong emotions that result from these conversations. In response to their discomfort, physicians frequently present information in an overly optimistic manner when discussing prognosis and avoid direct questions about death. Families share that receiving honest prognostic information from their provider and having the opportunity to discuss death in a compassionate manner does not remove hope.[32] Medical decision-making is an expression of family values and beliefs combined with an understanding of medical information.[31]

END-OF-LIFE CARE

Childhood mortality has remained stable for the past 50 years, with most childhood deaths occurring in those younger than 1 year. Hospital-based deaths remain the most common, with nearly three-quarters occurring in an ICU.[33] The primary manner of death has become the withdrawal of life-sustaining technology.[34] Children in the United States die in far fewer numbers in the emergency department, operating room, inpatient ward, hospice center, and at home. In any setting, the primary goal is to ensure the comfort of the child and the family.

Voicing My Choices and Five Wishes

Planning for the death of a child, adolescent, or young adult is difficult. Many worry that open conversations will diminish hope and thus do not offer those dying a forum for supported conversation. Respect for patient autonomy is a fundamental ethical principle in medicine. Children are considered to have diminished decision-making capacity, so their parents or legal guardians are identified as the persons best able to act in the child's best interest. A minor child can participate in creating an advanced directive. Children can provide input to their parent or legal guardian who is completing one or they can create their own. Although their own document will not be legally binding, it can give older children the opportunity to express what they are thinking and feeling and can help parents and caregivers when they are making decisions.

Voicing My Choices is a planning guide created for adolescents and young adults facing the end of their lives. It is a workbook that provides sentence starters and choices through check boxes on topics such as the following: ways I want to be comforted, ways I want to be supported, treatments I want, how I want to be remembered, and what I want done with my belongings after I die. Five Wishes is a similar guide useful for those older than 18 years. These documents can help families and providers start difficult end-of-life conversations, honor their dying child, and reinforce trusting relationships based on respect. These documents do allow for naming of a health care proxy and establishing resuscitation decisions that may be legally binding on a state-by-state basis. Often the next step is to complete a formal Medical Order of Life-Sustaining Treatment (MOLST).

More than half of the states in the United States have no statutes specifically addressing end-of-life decisions by minors. Some states recognize "emancipated minors" or have "minor treatment" statutes that provide for legal competency to be recognized in specific individuals younger than 18 years and/or in certain situations for patients younger than 18 years. "Emancipated minors" statutes recognize the autonomy of individuals on the basis of marriage, parenthood, financial independence, and other circumstances. "Minor treatment" statutes permit minors to authorize treatment for medical conditions they might not attend to if their parents were to know about them (sexually transmitted infections, pregnancy, and substance abuse). Under the "mature minor doctrine" some states have authorized judicial hearings in specific situations to grant capable adolescents the authority to decide for themselves about recommended medical therapy, sometimes against their parents' views[35]

Children's and younger adolescents' preferences should be considered seriously while maintaining final authority with an adult caregiver.[35,36] Early and open communication with caregivers regarding the health care provider's responsibility to the pediatric patient (ie, physicians are obligated to tell the truth to the child or adolescent if directly asked about dying), and because nondisclosure can interfere with a child's/adolescent's preparatory work before dying, must take place to avoid situations in which important information is kept from the patient.

CONCURRENT CARE AND HOSPICE

Hospice is a philosophy in which care focuses on the quality of a person's life and the person's comfort, independent of the length of life. Hospice care is provided by multidisciplinary teams whose care is often centered in the child's home. They provide an extra layer of support for persons for whom death can be expected within the next 6 months if the disease runs its normal course. Children (those younger than 21 years) are eligible to receive the support of hospice services while pursuing disease-modifying therapies. Having the ability to enroll children with hospice teams allows for a greater range of services to be provided from the home. Oftentimes families will choose to have their child stay at home through death and thus can be supported with the help of a hospice team.

THE DYING CHILD

Cognitive development plays a role in a child's understanding of death. At a young age, death may be viewed as temporary and associated with old age. As children get older they develop magical thinking and may believe that death is their fault. By age 7, most children understand that death is irreversible and they become interested in talking about death. As children become older they also consider the effect that death has on the people around them. Children with terminal illness often are aware of their imminent death.[37] Many children have an accelerated level of maturity due to the experience of living with a chronic or terminal illness and that reflects in an advanced understanding of their own end of life.[38] Parents frequently regret their decision not to discuss death with their dying child.[38] It is natural for parents to be protective of their child and refrain from talking about difficult and painful issues. Social workers, art therapists, and child life therapists can help with preparing for, starting, or having this conversation. Children can develop anxiety and mistrust when they are left out of important conversations, especially when it pertains to them.[39] Open-ended questions can help to appreciate what the child understands. Clarifying their questions is essential, as their concept of death can range from totally erroneous to magical to extremely concrete. Using language that is appropriate for the developmental stage of the child is essential.[39] Concrete language with younger children is necessary to avoid confusion and unnecessary fear.

The dying process is a time to help prepare the patient and family members, including siblings, for a future without the child. There are many different elements to consider, such as medical management of physical and psychological symptoms, as well as preparing to support the family and patient. Because the death of a child within the hospital is an infrequent occurrence, it is useful to develop a checklist that staff can refer to in order to support families through this difficult time. Institutional-specific contact information should be included as well (**Box 2**).

Box 2
End-of-life checklist

Environment
☐ Lighting (soft, adjustable)
☐ Sound (monitors with volume decreased, music)
☐ Beverages, tissues
☐ Privacy screens and signage to alert that death is impending/has occurred

Support
☐ Interpreter: in person or by phone/video
☐ Clergy/religious community invited to be present, perform rituals
☐ Sibling visitation opportunities with the assistance of child life or social work
☐ Space for family in the patient room or outside

Memory Making
☐ Handprints/molds or fingerprint charm
☐ Bathing and dressing of child
☐ Memory box
☐ Photography

Logistics
☐ Contact organ procurement organization before death occurs to facilitate screening for organ and tissue donation
☐ Discuss autopsy services
☐ Declaration of time of death
☐ Contact medical examiner
☐ Completion of death certificate

BEREAVEMENT

The death of a child has a profound impact on the entire family. The parent-child relationship is unique, and a child's death evokes feelings of inadequacy and failure in addition to the typical emotional responses of anger, anxiety, sadness, loneliness, and fear. Grandparents suffer their own loss and grieve for the loss that their child is suffering as well. Siblings experience a loss of their sibling, a loss of the family unit, and a loss of the caregivers to the grief process.

Families of deceased children have indicated that continued contact with staff after their child's death was meaningful to them; follow-up may be by telephone, mail, and/ or in person.[12] Parents also note that certain experiences with the health care staff perceived as painful by the parents can interfere with their long-term grieving process.[12] Specifically, insensitive delivery of bad news, feeling dismissed or patronized, perceived disregard for parents' judgment regarding care of their child, and poor communication of important information were found to disturb family members and complicate grief years later.[12] When a child dies, it is a profound loss for the family, health care team, and community (**Box 3**).

Box 3
Top books for children/families

When Dinosaurs Die: A Guide to Understanding Death by Laurie Krasny Brown and Marc Brown. Little Brown and Company 2009

A Terrible Thing Happened by Margaret M. Holmes. Magination Press 2000

The Invisible String by Patrice Karst. DeVorss Publications 2000

The Healing Book; Facing the death and celebrating the life of someone you love by Ellen Sabin. Watering Can Press 2006

Help Me Say Goodbye: Activities for Helping Kids Cope When A Special Person Dies by Janis Silverman. Fairview Press 1999

Brother: A Grief Story by Teleah Scott-Williams. Mascot-Books 2013.

Be the Boss of Your Pain by Timothy Culbert and Rebecca Kajander. Free Spirit Publishing 2007

Be the Boss of Your Stress by Timothy Culbert and Rebecca Kajander. Free Spirit Publishing 2007

SUMMARY

Caring for children and their families facing serious illness requires a team approach. Providing attention to emotional, physical, social, and spiritual pain will lessen the burden of suffering. When caring for children, you are caring for the future hopes of an entire family, and when a child dies everyone is impacted uniquely. Advocating for early involvement with palliative care is always appropriate to ensure that each child has the chance to live their best day.

REFERENCES

1. Lemmon ME, Bidegain M, Boss RD. Palliative care in neonatal neurology: robust support for infants, families and clinicians. J Perinatol 2016;36(5):331–7.
2. Ammentorp J, Mainz J, Sabroe S. Parents' priorities and satisfaction with acute pediatric care. Arch Pediatr Adolesc Med 2005;159(2):127–31.
3. Bieri D, Reeve RA, Champion GD, et al. The Faces Pain Scale for the self-assessment of the severity of pain experienced by children: development, initial validation, and preliminary investigation for ratio scale properties. Pain 1990; 41(2):139–50.
4. Beyer J. The oucher: a user's manual and technical report. Evanston (IL): Judson Press; 1984. p. 1–12.
5. Hauer J, Houtrow AJ, Section on Hospice and Palliative Medicine, Council on Children with Disabilities. Pain assessment and treatment in children with significant impairment of the central nervous system. Pediatrics 2017;139(6) [pii: e20171002].
6. Markman JD, Philip A. Interventional approaches to pain management. Anesthesiol Clin 2007;25(4):883–98, viii.

7. Friedrichsdorf SJ, Kang TI. The management of pain in children with life-limiting illnesses. Pediatr Clin North Am 2007;54(5):645–72, x.

8. Sahler OJ, Frager G, Levetown M, et al. Medical education about end-of-life care in the pediatric setting: principles, challenges, and opportunities. Pediatrics 2000;105(3 Pt 1):575–84.

9. Cassileth BR. Complementary and alternative cancer medicine. J Clin Oncol 1999;17(11 Suppl):44–52.

10. Moody K, Abrahams B, Baker R, et al. A Randomized Trial of Yoga for Children Hospitalized With Sickle Cell Vaso-Occlusive Crisis. J Pain Symptom Manage 2017;53(6):1026–34.

11. Tsao JC, Zeltzer LK. Complementary and alternative medicine approaches for pediatric pain: a review of the state-of-the-science. Evid Based Complement Alternat Med 2005;2(2):149–59.

12. Gottschling S, Reindl TK, Meyer S, et al. Acupuncture to alleviate chemotherapy-induced nausea and vomiting in pediatric oncology - a randomized multicenter crossover pilot trial. Klin Padiatr 2008;220(6):365–70.

13. Ladas EJ, Post-White J, Hawks R, et al. Evidence for symptom management in the child with cancer. J Pediatr Hematol Oncol 2006;28(9):601–15.

14. Patel AK, Bell MJ, Traube C. Delirium in pediatric critical care. Pediatr Clin North Am 2017;64(5):1117–32.

15. Keele L, Keenan HT, Sheetz J, et al. Differences in characteristics of dying children who receive and do not receive palliative care. Pediatrics 2013;132(1):72–8.

16. Wolfe J, Grier HE, Klar N, et al. Symptoms and suffering at the end of life in children with cancer. N Engl J Med 2000;342(5):326–33.

17. Maslow GR, Dunlap K, Chung RJ. Depression and suicide in children and adolescents. Pediatr Rev 2015;36(7):299–308 [quiz: 309–310].

18. Hedstrom M, Kreuger A, Ljungman G, et al. Accuracy of assessment of distress, anxiety, and depression by physicians and nurses in adolescents recently diagnosed with cancer. Pediatr Blood Cancer 2006;46(7):773–9.

19. Shemesh E, Annunziato RA, Shneider BL, et al. Parents and clinicians underestimate distress and depression in children who had a transplant. Pediatr Transplant 2005;9(5):673–9.

20. Kovacs M. The children's depression inventory (CDI). Psychopharmacol Bull 1985;21(4):995–8.

21. Collins JJ, Devine TD, Dick GS, et al. The measurement of symptoms in young children with cancer: the validation of the Memorial Symptom Assessment Scale in children aged 7-12. J Pain Symptom Manage 2002;23(1):10–6.

22. Kersun LS, Shemesh E. Depression and anxiety in children at the end of life. Pediatr Clin North Am 2007;54(5):691–708, xi.

23. Tang MH, Pinsky EG. Mood and affect disorders. Pediatr Rev 2015;36(2):52–60 [quiz: 61].

24. Fitchett G, Lyndes KA, Cadge W, et al. The role of professional chaplains on pediatric palliative care teams: perspectives from physicians and chaplains. J Palliat Med 2011;14(6):704–7.

25. Kelly JA, May CS, Maurer SH. Assessment of the spiritual needs of primary caregivers of children with life-limiting illnesses is valuable yet inconsistently performed in the hospital. J Palliat Med 2016;19(7):763–6.

26. Hexem KR, Mollen CJ, Carroll K, et al. How parents of children receiving pediatric palliative care use religion, spirituality, or life philosophy in tough times. J Palliat Med 2011;14(1):39–44.

27. Sadof M, Gortakowski M, Stechenberg B, et al. The "HEADS AT" training tool for residents: a roadmap for caring for children with medical complexity. Clin Pediatr (Phila) 2015;54(12):1210–4.
28. Muscara F, Burke K, McCarthy MC, et al. Parent distress reactions following a serious illness or injury in their child: a protocol paper for the take a Breath Cohort Study. BMC Psychiatry 2015;15:153.
29. Carroll C, Carroll C, Goloff N, et al. When bad news isn't necessarily bad: recognizing provider bias when sharing unexpected news. Pediatrics 2018;142(1) [pii: e20180503].
30. Feudtner C, Walter JK, Faerber JA, et al. Good-parent beliefs of parents of seriously ill children. JAMA Pediatr 2015;169(1):39–47.
31. Tucker Edmonds B, Torke AM, Helft P, et al. Doctor, what would you do? An ANSWER for patients requesting advice about value-laden decisions. Pediatrics 2015;136(4):740–5.
32. Bernacki RE, Block SD, American College of Physicians High Value Care Task Force. Communication about serious illness care goals: a review and synthesis of best practices. JAMA Intern Med 2014;174(12):1994–2003.
33. Leyenaar JK, Bogetz JF. Child mortality in the United States: bridging palliative care and public health perspectives. Pediatrics 2018;142(4) [pii:e20181927].
34. Trowbridge A, Walter JK, McConathey E, et al. Modes of death within a children's hospital. Pediatrics 2018;142(4) [pii:e20174182].
35. Freyer DR. Care of the dying adolescent: special considerations. Pediatrics 2004; 113(2):381–8.
36. Hinds PS, Drew D, Oakes LL, et al. End-of-life care preferences of pediatric patients with cancer. J Clin Oncol 2005;23(36):9146–54.
37. Black D. The dying child. BMJ 1998;316(7141):1376–8.
38. Kushnick HL. Trusting them with the truth-disclosure and the good death for children with terminal illness. Virtual Mentor 2010;12(7):573–7.
39. Bates AT, Kearney JA. Understanding death with limited experience in life: dying children's and adolescents' understanding of their own terminal illness and death. Curr Opin Support Palliat Care 2015;9(1):40–5.

Moving?

Make sure your subscription moves with you!

To notify us of your new address, find your **Clinics Account Number** (located on your mailing label above your name), and contact customer service at:

Email: journalscustomerservice-usa@elsevier.com

800-654-2452 (subscribers in the U.S. & Canada)
314-447-8871 (subscribers outside of the U.S. & Canada)

Fax number: 314-447-8029

Elsevier Health Sciences Division
Subscription Customer Service
3251 Riverport Lane
Maryland Heights, MO 63043

*To ensure uninterrupted delivery of your subscription, please notify us at least 4 weeks in advance of move.

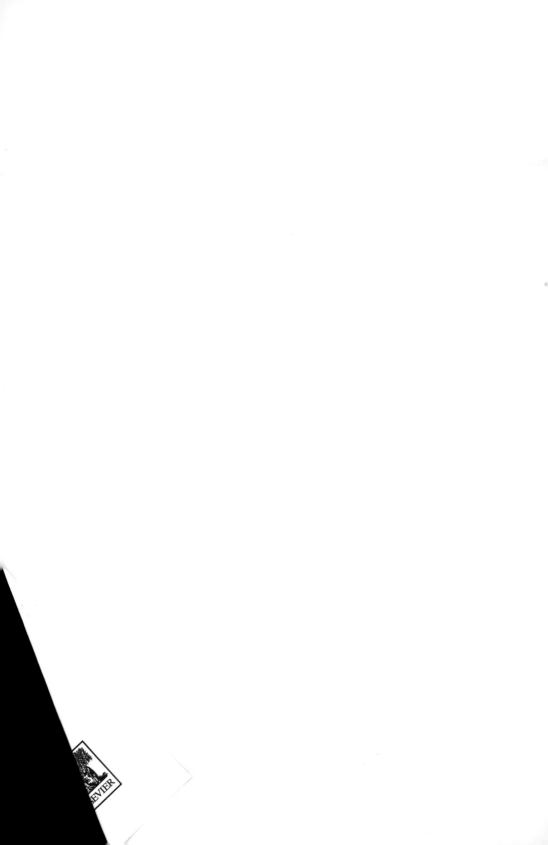